GET WELL SOON

GET WELL SOON

History's Worst Plagues and the Heroes Who Fought Them

JENNIFER WRIGHT

Henry Holt and Company
New York

Henry Holt and Company
Publishers since 1866
175 Fifth Avenue
New York, New York 10010
www.henryholt.com

Henry Holt® and 🐝® are registered trademarks of Macmillan Publishing Group, LLC.

Library of Congress Cataloging-in-Publication Data

Names: Wright, Jennifer Ashley, 1986- author.
Title: Get well soon : history's worst plagues and the heroes who fought them
    / by Jennifer Wright.
Description: First edition. | New York : Henry Holt and Company, 2017. |
    Includes bibliographical references.
Identifiers: LCCN 2016029515| ISBN 9781627797467 (hardback) | ISBN
    9781627797474 (electronic book)
Subjects: LCSH: Epidemics—History. | Communicable diseases—History. |
    Epidemiology—Social aspects. | BISAC: HISTORY / Essays. | HISTORY /
    Social History.
Classification: LCC RA649 .W75 2017 | DDC 614.4—dc23
LC record available at https://lccn.loc.gov/2016029515

Our books may be purchased in bulk for promotional, educational, or business use.
Please contact your local bookseller or the Macmillan Corporate and Premium Sales
Department at (800) 221-7945, extension 5442, or by e-mail at MacmillanSpecialMarkets@
macmillan.com.

First Edition 2017

Designed by Meryl Sussman Levavi

Printed in the United States of America

10   9   8   7   6   5   4

For Mom and Dad.
Would it kill you to go to the doctor now
and then?

What's natural is the microbe. All the rest—health,
integrity, purity (if you like)—is a product of the human
will, of a vigilance that must never falter.

—ALBERT CAMUS, *The Plague*

I've got chills.
They're multiplying.
And I'm losing control.

—JOHN FARRAR,
"You're the One That I Want," *Grease*

Contents

GET WELL SOON

Introduction

When I tell people that I am writing a book on plagues, well-meaning acquaintances suggest I add a modern twist. Specifically: "You know, like how we're all on our cell phones all the time." Or selfies. A chapter on selfies.

Then I reply, "No, my interest lies more with the kind of plague where you break out in sores all over your body and countless people you know and love die, rapidly, within a few months of each other, in the prime of their lives. And there is nothing you can do, and everyone is dead, and everything is death, and all of earth seems to be a vast wasteland of corpses, and, wait, here, allow me to show you some absolutely horrific pictures."

And then they say, "Excuse me, I'm just going to get another drink."

I am so happy you picked up this book because often, when

I'm out chatting with people, no one really likes to hear about diseases of the past. I suspect that disinclination is largely due to plagues seeming both very grim and very remote. It's generally better just to say that I like selfies. I think they're fun. I like seeing pictures of my friends' smiling faces. I like how alive they all are.

It does appear that we are living in a world where the word *plague* has shockingly little meaning for many. To the extent that they think about plagues at all, many associate them with muddy huts, textbooks they had to read in sixth grade, and, if they are film buffs, a death figure who has a truly bewildering interest in chess. People in core countries seem to expect to die at age ninety in a nursing home. They do so with good reason: if conditions continue uninterrupted, 50 percent of the children born in the year 2000 will live to be a hundred years old.

If conditions continue uninterrupted.

We have been living in an age of improbable luck. We have experienced nearly thirty years without a disease—that we do not know how to combat—killing upward of thousands of otherwise healthy young people in those core countries. I can't say whether this good fortune will run out—I hope it won't—but it always has in the past. We just like to forget this disagreeable fact. Forgetting is soothing and probably in our nature. But disregarding, and being ignorant of, plagues of the past makes us more, rather than less, vulnerable to inevitable ones in the future.

Because when plagues erupt, some people behave amazingly well. They minimize the level of death and destruction around them. They are kind. They are courageous. They showcase the best of our nature.

Other people behave like superstitious lunatics and add to the death toll.

I wish I had the scientific knowledge to talk about how to make vaccines or cures that might eradicate illness, but I don't.

This book isn't just for future Nobel Prize winners, as much as I am impressed by and rooting for them. Because whether plagues are managed quickly doesn't just depend on hardworking doctors and scientists. It depends on people who like to sleep in on weekends and watch movies and eat French fries and do the fantastic common things in life, which is to say, it depends on all of us. Whether a civilization fares well during a crisis has a great deal to do with how the ordinary, nonscientist citizen responds. A lot of the measures taken against the plagues discussed in this book will seem stunningly obvious. You should not, for instance, decide diseased people are sinners and burn them at a literal or metaphorical stake, because it is both morally monstrous and entirely ineffective. Everyone would probably theoretically agree with this statement. But then a new plague crops up, and we make precisely the same mistakes we should have learned from three hundred years ago.

I recently read in a history book that you ought not view the past through a modern-day lens. It supposed that instead you should consider different eras as entirely separate, like, I imagine, sausage links. I thought the writer seemed to show a fundamental lack of understanding of how time works. The past does not exist under a bell jar. Moments, ideas, and tragedies of the past bleed into the present. Alas, some of the ideas that make it into the present consciousness are not the best. I found, for instance, that some people still feel justified hating Jews because they think they started the bubonic plague by dumping diseased material into wells. (This is, as we'll examine, impossible.) Worrying whether people preparing your food are washing their hands thoroughly has a lot to do with the contagious disease-carrying cook Mary Mallon, aka Typhoid Mary. If moments from the past seep so seamlessly into the present, maybe moments from the present can help us relate to the past. After all, the past was no less ridiculous than the present. Both eras were made up of humans.

One of my great wishes is that people of the present will see those of the past as friendly (or irritating) acquaintances they can look to for advice. It's easy to forget that people from the past weren't the two-dimensional black-and-white photos or line drawings you might encounter in some dry textbooks. They weren't just gray-faced guys in top hats. They were living, breathing, joking, burping people, who could be happy or sad, funny or boring, cool or the lamest people you ever met in your life. They had no idea they were living in the past. They all thought they were living in the present. Accordingly, like any person, past or present, could be, some of them were smart and kind and geniuses about medicine and also completely dull on a personal level. (I'm trying to come to terms with loving John Snow's deductive brilliance and being absolutely certain I would never want to spend more than ten minutes talking to him.) Others were charismatic and charming and total sociopathic maniacs. (That description gives Walter Jackson Freeman II too much credit for charm, but people liked him. He was gross, and he wore a weird penis ring on his neck. People should not have liked him for numerous reasons.)

You should regard everyone in this book as human, not inanimate *historical figures*. We can have personal opinions about them; we're not all that different from them. And despite what some breathtakingly stupid intellectuals would have you believe, the people and interests of the past weren't necessarily smart and serious any more than the people and interests of the present are dumb and frivolous. Knowing about pop culture doesn't make you dumb; it makes you a person who is interested in the world you live in. Besides, it is impossible to believe that everyone in the past was a serious figure meriting great respect once you learn that one guy thought tubercular patients should take up new careers as alligator hunters.

I am always hopeful that the more we demystify the past—and the more we laugh about it and toss around information about it with the same enthusiasm we have for discussing our favorite TV shows—the better off we will be. Because if or when the next plague comes, I hate the idea that the only people who are familiar with Paracelsus (loved mercury, hated women) are going to be elderly academics in tweed coats who discuss him with pseudo-British accents. When the next outbreak comes—and I lack the optimism to believe it won't—so many of our challenges will remain the same. We will be so much better off if the absolute maximum number of present-day and future people handle the disease with the aplomb of some of the best figures in this book. And let's be honest, that guy in the tweed coat with the on-again-off-again accent is going to die first.

I'm invested in this study of diseases because I think knowing how diseases have been combatted in the past will be helpful in the future. If you're someone who intends on living into the future, I hope you will be, too.

And don't worry. You don't need to flee for another drink. I'll keep the horrific pictures to a minimum. Despite the considerable odds against it, I'll try to make reading and learning about these dark times in human history a lot of fun.

Antonine Plague

*When you arise in the morning,
think of what a precious privilege it
is to be alive—to breathe, to think, to
enjoy, to love.*

—MARCUS AURELIUS

Every so often—frequently when consenting adults are reported to be having sex in some manner that would have been banned in the Victorian age—a TV commentator will shake his head and discuss how this behavior led to Rome's final days. Often it seems those pundits have a poor understanding of kindness, compassion for one's fellow man, and the progressive flow of social mores. And we can absolutely say they always have a poor grasp of "Rome's final days."

To be clear, the Roman Empire didn't end because everybody was having sex. No civilization was ever toppled by "too much sexy time"—except for Bavaria in 1848, but that is an unrelated (if delightful) story.

The beginning of the final days of Rome wasn't caused by heartwarming weddings between gay people. It began with a plague that erupted in the 160s. At that very time Romans were at the height of their power and their massive empire stretched from Scotland to Syria.

They were able to conquer and defend such a huge empire because the Roman army was a massive force. During the period around 160, the army consisted of twenty-eight legions composed of 5,120 men each. The legionnaires volunteered to serve for twenty-five years, after which time they could retire with a generous pension of about fourteen years' pay. And in case 143,360 men in the army seems a little light—for comparison there are currently approximately 520,000 active duty soldiers in the United States—there were additional auxiliary armies that made up about another 60 percent of the force. Those were often composed of noncitizens who, if they survived their years of service, were granted Roman citizenship.

Now, you may wonder, *Yes, but who would survive twenty-five years in the military?* If you were a Roman soldier, your chances of staying alive during the period 135 to 160 were actually comparatively reasonable. While the exact statistics are unknown, it was a time of relatively few battles. You might not even have to fight. Walter Scheidel, a professor at Stanford University, writes: "For all we can tell, the 239 veterans (representing two years' worth of releases) who were discharged from legio[n] VII Claudia around AD 160 had not experienced substantial combat operations during their twenty-five or twenty-six years of service."[1]

Those troops didn't see action in *twenty-five years*. I bet they were laughingstocks. But that's a good thing! They did not have to fight, ever!

If they did see battle, the Roman troops were stunningly, perhaps even unnecessarily, well equipped. The legionnaires were outfitted with lorica segmentata, an extremely flexible armor made of metal strips. The first-century historian Josephus described the impressively arrayed Roman army: "They march forward, everyone silent and in correct order, each man maintaining his particular position in the ranks, just as he would in battle. The infantry are equipped with breastplates and helmets and carry a sword on both sides. The infantry chosen to guard the general carry a javelin and an oblong sword. However, they also carry a saw, a basket, a shovel, and an ax, as well as a leather strap, a scythe, a chain, and three days' food rations."[2] They were like the Swiss army knives of soldiers.

So the Roman army had great armor, great numbers, great training, and in some cases at least three days of food on them at all times. Shortly after this, they'd begin losing battles and cities to the Germanic tribes.

I initially thought that the Germanic tribes must have had some fairly cool equipment to successfully combat the Imperial Roman army. Fortunately, Tacitus was there to set me straight. The Germanic tribes fighting them were pretty much naked. The historian wrote of at least one Germanic tribe: "They are either naked, or lightly covered with a small mantle; and have no pride in equipage: their shields only are ornamented with the choicest colors. Few are provided with a coat of mail and scarcely here and there one with a casque or helmet."[3] I especially like that Tacitus took time to scoff that the German shields were artistically weak. The *Encyclopedia Britannica*, in an instance of unusually helpful specificity, backs up Tacitus, explaining that the Germanic tribes would all be horribly ill equipped until the sixth century:

Their chief weapon was a long lance, and few carried swords. Helmets and breastplates were almost unknown. A light wooden or wicker shield, sometimes fitted with an iron rim and sometimes strengthened with leather, was the only defensive weapon. This lack of adequate equipment explains the swift, fierce rush with which the Germans would charge the ranks of the heavily armed Romans. If they became entangled in a prolonged, hand-to-hand grapple, where their light shields and thrusting spears were confronted with Roman swords and armour, they had little hope of success.[4]

In spite of their inferior equipment the tribes were *incredibly* courageous. Women fought alongside men, sometimes with their children. For many, their greatest wish was to die a glorious death in battle. The nineteenth-century historian John George Sheppard describes the German tribes: "Though often defeated, they were never conquered; a wave might roll back, but the tide advanced; they held firmly to their purpose till it was attained; they wrested the ball and sceptre from Roman hands, and have kept them until now."[5] The Germanic tribes were willing to continually attack the Roman Empire despite being outnumbered and possessing inferior armor and weaponry. They were ready. They lived for battle. They had been threatening, though failing to penetrate, the empire's borders since being defeated by the Roman general Gaius Marius in 101 BC. I'm not saying that it was surprising that they attacked. I am saying they never should have won. The best army in the world still, logically, shouldn't have been defeated by a bunch of nearly naked people with presumably taupe-colored shields.

But the tribes had the strongest ally in the world on their side. It wasn't human. It was the Antonine plague.

The expanse of territory the Roman troops covered would prove to be their undoing This plague came to Rome from Mesopotamia around AD 165–66. It was carried home by Roman troops who had been fighting in that region. And when it arrived in Rome it was a *nightmare*. A nightmare even by the standards of people who were used to disease.

Although we may rave about how technologically advanced Rome seemed compared to the Dark Ages following Roman civilization's collapse, it was imperfect. There were public latrines, but few private houses were connected to public sewers; many people dumped their waste directly onto the streets. The Tiber River was also prone to flooding, which meant (forgive this description but there's no other clear way to say it) that a river of shit would occasionally flow through the streets. And though people used bathhouses, the water they bathed in wasn't disinfected and frequently contained bacteria. As you might expect, malaria, typhoid, dysentery, hepatitis, and cholera all thrived during the period, yet the historian Edward Gibbon claimed this was the age during which, "the human race was most happy and prosperous." I should cut Gibbon a little slack here—he published his *Decline and Fall of the Roman Empire* beginning in 1776—but pretending any historical age before proper indoor plumbing was a glorious epoch is a ludicrous delusion. Frank McLynn, a modern-day historian, writes in *Marcus Aurelius, A Life*: "Horrific as malaria and all the other deadly diseases were, Romans absorbed them as part of daily existence; slaves and other wretched of the Earth were already living a death-in-life, so they may not have been unduly perturbed by the approach of the Reaper. But the 'plague' that hit Rome under Marcus Aurelius was entirely different, both in degree and kind, from anything Romans had experienced before."[6]

Much of what we know about the nature of this plague is taken from the writings of Marcus Aurelius's physician, Galen. In fact, the Antonine plague is even sometimes called the Plague of Galen.

Although Galen was a great physician, he was not a terribly courageous man. Galen was a self-promoter above anything else. According to McLynn, he consistently claimed to be a self-made man, casually downplaying the fact that he came from an extremely wealthy family and had inherited numerous estates as well as a stellar list of contacts. He employed underhanded tactics to win debates, and he constantly aggrandized his own

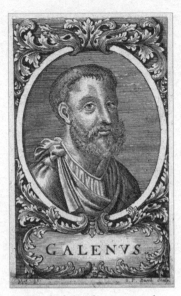

GALENVS

Tiny little hands not pictured.

achievements. Personality-wise, you could think of him as the Donald Trump of ancient Rome. He was also something of a coward when it came to disease. Now, I don't think cowardice is an abnormal reaction in life-or-death situations; it can be very similar to intelligent self-preservation. I fully expect that I would be weak and spineless in a plague. However, it's not a great trait in a physician.

Galen came very close to not recording this plague at all. When the disease began breaking out in 166, he fled Rome for the less disease-ridden countryside. He claimed he was leaving Rome not because he was understandably scared, but because all the other physicians were so jealous of him and his awesome skills that Rome just wasn't a cool place to be anymore. We don't know exactly where he was from 166 to 168, only that he was summoned back to join Marcus Aurelius in Aquileia (today northern Adriatic Italy) in 168. One year later, when the outbreak worsened in that region, Galen told Marcus Aurelius that the Greco-Roman god of medicine Asclepius had come to him in a dream and said that Galen should go home to Rome *for sure*. Galen claimed the god regularly chatted with him in his dreams and gave him advice on a number of medical matters. I don't put it past Galen to use an "a god told me to do it" excuse to remove himself from danger, but it's also possible that he did believe these messages. Marcus Aurelius mercifully allowed Galen to return to Rome, where he spent the rest of his life as the private physician to the future emperor Commodus. He lived, seemingly very happily, into his eighties—a major accomplishment considering the generally shortened life spans of his era.

Fortunately for us, despite his best efforts, Galen didn't succeed in avoiding the pestilence entirely. Instead, he studied and wrote extensively about the Antonine plague. From his records we know specifics about the symptoms and progression of the disease. We know that the plague caused victims to break out, very suddenly, in small red spots all over their bodies, and after one or two days, the spots would turn into a rash. Fever blisters would then swell for the next two weeks, before scabbing over and breaking off, leaving an ashy appearance all over the body. We also know that victims would develop a fever, though perhaps not one that was immediately obvious. Galen wrote: "Those afflicted with the plague appear neither warm nor burning to those who touch them, although they are raging with fever inside, just as Thucydides describes."[7]

Galen's remarks upon Thucydides's description are most likely in reference to the latter's devastating account of the Plague of Athens in 430 BC, which wiped out around two-thirds of Athens's population. Galen might have understandably thought the two afflictions were one and the same. I love that Galen was just casually familiar with a text written six hundred years before his time! Reading history books is great! However, the two plagues don't have much in common other than victims developing a high fever and then dying. Today, the Plague of Athens is usually thought to have been bubonic plague or possibly the ebola virus, whereas modern physicians suspect the Antonine plague was smallpox.

Still, it is interesting that Thucydides is referenced, because the Plague of Athens was regarded as an apocalyptic event. Thucydides writes:

> Mortality raged without restraint. The bodies of dying men lay one upon another, and half-dead creatures reeled about

the streets and gathered round all the fountains in their long-
ing for water. The sacred places also in which they had quar-
tered themselves were full of corpses of persons that had died
there, just as they were; for as the disaster passed all bounds,
men, not knowing what was to become of them, became
utterly careless of everything, whether sacred or profane.[8]

By comparing the two, Galen gives a sense of the magnitude
of the Antonine plague—unless he is wildly hyperbolic. Given
his personality, I can see how that might give one pause. But
although Galen was a showboater, he wasn't deliberately in-
accurate about anything except the greatness of his own skills.

Galen is less interested in the historical and societal impact
of "his" plague than Thucydides was. His writings focus instead
on how certain ailments progressed and what factors might
indicate a patient's potential survival. Galen writes: "Black excrement was a symptom of those who had the disease, whether
they survived or perished of it . . . if the stool was not black, the
exanthem always appeared. All those who excreted black stool
died of it."[9] This kind of writing is *great*. This is one of the first
times in the historical record that a figure writes about a disease
as a physician rather than as a historian. Doubtless that information was of great interest to anyone who was tending to a loved
one, insofar as if their feces turned black, you would know to
start making funeral arrangements.

Today, experts turn to Galen's writings to determine the
precise nature of the plague. Through the precision of his descriptions, we know that about two weeks after the first symptoms
of the Antonine plague (the blisters), a rash would begin to coat
the tongue and throat of the afflicted. Galen also noted that
many victims coughed up blood. He describes one man as vomiting up scabs, which is maybe the foulest image I can give you.

As horrible as the disease sounds, not everyone died from
it. If you had what Galen called "black exanthema" (which

means a "breaking out" or a widespread rash), you had a good likelihood of surviving. Galen even tells, happily, of a man rising from his bed on the twelfth day of the disease. He claims:

> On those who would survive who had diarrhea, a black exanthema appeared on the whole body. Due to a remnant of blood, which had putrefied in the fever blisters, like some ash that nature had deposited on the body. Of some of those who became ulcerated, the part of the surface called the scab fell away and then the remaining part nearby was healthy and after one or two days became scarred over. In those places where it was not ulcerated the exanthema was rough and scabby and fell away like some husk and hence all became healthy.[10]

There's debate today over whether the plague that led to Rome's fall was typhus or measles or smallpox. I am on Team Smallpox!

However, no matter which disease it was, the debate would have made no difference to anyone at the time. There was no medicine that would come close to treating any of them. Before 1600, people would have difficulty differentiating any type of disease from another; any quickly spreading epidemic would simply be referred to as a plague.

Scholars also continue to debate over the total death toll from the Antonine plague. Frank McLynn notes, "Even if we split the difference between the most impressive scholarly studies, we can't get lower than a total mortality of 10 million."[11] It was probably higher! McLynn himself estimates the total death toll as around 18 million. At the height of the outbreak, slightly later in 189, Cassius Dio claimed it caused around two thousand deaths a day in Rome. There's certainly no estimate that makes the death toll from this plague anything short of overwhelming.

I'd love to tell you about how the disease was treated, cured, or even prevented with any degree of effectiveness. But I can't! It was the year 166, and that optimism is reserved for future chapters in history. The Roman people may have prayed for a cure, but the best they could hope for was someone who was able to keep society minimally functional. Because if you are a citizen of any time, you really don't want a repeat of the Plague of Athens, where corpses were piling up in the temples. In almost every plague throughout history, it takes a remarkably strong leader just to keep the bodies out of the streets.

Rome was fortunate. That leader was Marcus Aurelius, the last of those described by Machiavelli as the Five Good Emperors. Beyond being the emperor who employed Galen, Marcus Aurelius practiced a philosophy you're probably familiar with: Stoicism. If not, some freshman taking Philosophy 101 is going to tell you about it with great excitement one of these days. I will preempt that student by saying that the basic tenet of Stoicism is to exercise reason and employ restraint over emotions, especially the negative ones like anger and greed. One should attempt to behave in accordance with nature, accepting and being prepared for the unchangeable aspects of existence, such as death. The philosophy is beautifully summarized by Marcus Aurelius in his *Meditations*: "Say to yourself in the early morning: I shall meet today inquisitive, ungrateful, violent, treacherous, envious, uncharitable men. All of these things have come upon them through ignorance of real good and ill. But, because I have seen the nature of what is good and right, I can neither be harmed by any of them, for no man will involve me in wrong, nor can I be angry with my kinsman or hate him; for we have come into the world to work together."[12]

Stoics attempted to be guided by logic and reason rather than fleeting worldly pleasures. The practice of Stoicism supposedly allowed people to lead more peaceful, rational lives. Some citizens thought this philosophy made Marcus Aurelius hard to relate to, but, on the whole, Stoicism is straightforward and sensible, and the philosophy was popular. Certainly, it seems like it would be extremely useful in crisis situations.

I like to think that, across the ages, the Roman people considered this endorsement of Stoicism, collectively shook their heads, and responded, "Nah." As soon as the plague broke out, the population almost immediately abandoned calm, rational Stoicism in favor of believing in magic and killing Christians.

Hucksters like the mystic Alexander of Abonoteichos emerged selling useless charms for everyone to hang on their doorways. They contained simple protective sayings like "Long-haired Phoebus chases the cloud of pestilence."[13] Alexander became rich and famous. Of course he did. Charlatans preying upon people's fear with false hope during plague times often do. (This is the "career advice for sociopaths" portion of the book.)

When they weren't busy buying charms, people blamed the Christians for bringing the disease upon the city by angering the Olympian gods. This claim is absurd because anyone who has read *D'Aulaires' Book of Greek Myths* knows that Olympian gods' anger was more often expressed by "turning women into spiders as punishment for describing themselves as too beautiful" or "catching people in a net while having sex" rather than "raining down pustules and deadly disease over the empire." However, Christians were easy scapegoats. Marcus Aurelius already held Christians in contempt, regarding them as foolishly eager to rush into martyrdom. As a result, their treatment during his reign was so horrible it is referred to as "the Fourth Persecution" in *Foxe's Book of Martyrs*, which claims:

> Marcus Aurelius followed about the year of our Lord 161AD: a man of nature more stern and severe, and, although in the study of philosophy and civil government no less commendable, yet, towards the Christians sharp and fierce . . . The cruelties used in this persecution were such that many of the spectators shuddered with horror at the sight, and were

astonished at the intrepidity of the sufferers. Some of the martyrs were obliged to pass, with their already wounded feet, over thorns, nails, sharp shells, etc. upon their points, others were scourged until their sinews and veins lay bare, and after suffering the most excruciating tortures that could be devised, they were destroyed by the most terrible deaths.[14]

Persecuting religious minorities is always ill-advised, every single time it occurs in history. I have never in my research found an instance where a historian says, "Wow, we were on the right side of history for torturing Group X back then." Marcus Aurelius should have probably done something to protect these vulnerable citizens. But he didn't. He disliked them, *and* he had other pressing duties to contend with.

Aside from tacitly or overtly condoning the persecution of a religious sect, Marcus Aurelius responded to the plague with the kind of calm collection I think all of us should strive for while, say, on the phone with Time Warner Cable. He immediately busied himself signing new laws to keep the city livable. For instance, he forbade people from turning their villas into giant tombs. He excused anyone from a court summons who had a funeral to attend, and common people who died of the plague were given burials at the public's expense. A law was passed that you could not dig up bodies to use their graves for your own dead, which was apparently common enough to require legislation. All these laws were important, as undertakers were charging outrageous prices for the citizens' increasing need for burials, and, again, the main responsibility of a plague-time ruler is to stop bodies piling up in the streets. (Both because it's unsanitary and because it causes people to panic.)

More terrifying than the fatalities in cities was the fact that the army was afflicted and dying. Soldiers on furlough to visit their families later brought the disease back to camp with them, and they carried it to new legions. This led to a signifigant manpower shortage at an especially unfortunate time: the Germanic tribes had become increasingly restless and were attempting to cross the Danube.

By 167, Germanic tribes led by the Marcomanni advanced past the Roman borders. This was the first time Germanic tribes had successfully invaded the Italian peninsula in about 250 years. They razed Oderzo and proceeded to lay siege to Aquileia, one of the largest cities in the world at that time.

Marcus Aurelius went to the frontier. Under duress and in an attempt to replace the soldiers killed by the plague, he recruited just about anyone who could carry a sword to join the army.

That entailed recruiting gladiators, which seems like an obvious and excellent idea. Gladiators knew how to fight! They were very *good* at fighting. Unfortunately, this policy infuriated the people in Rome. They loved their gladiatorial games, and now, as if it weren't bad enough that their compatriots were dying in droves, Marcus Aurelius was sending their sports heroes away to fight on the border. The fact that few remained meant that gladiatorial matches became rarer and extremely expensive to attend. Society's need for "bread and circuses" doesn't go on hold when a plague surfaces. If anything, in uncertain and terrifying times people want *more* entertainment that allows them to escape reality. Marcus Aurelius dealt with the unrest by persuading authorities to force criminals already condemned to death to fight in the arena for the public's amusement, and promised the government would cover the cost of the spectacles. Marcus Aurelius also staged another, nonhuman-based amusement that featured hundreds of lions being shot by archers. Christians didn't fare well during these spectacles. The second-century scholar Tertullian recalled the resounding cry "Christianos ad leonem," which loosely translates as "throw the Christians to the lions!" That is horrific. However, these methods satisfied the public bloodlust while the trained gladiators continued to defend the borders.

Marcus Aurelius also recruited bandits, offering them a

bounty to join the army. He enlisted freed slaves and even rival Germanic tribesmen for the army. Now, the problems with bandits are obvious: they are outlaws and may not be great at following the strict rules of an army. The problems with enlisting Teutonic people had more to do with how the Roman soldiers would respond to them. Enlisting freed slaves may seem less troublesome, but many of them had been granted liberty because they had grown old and their masters no longer wanted to spend money on their caretaking. Marcus Aurelius basically turned the once-formidable Roman army into the Night's Watch from the television show *Game of Thrones* (2011 to present).

Given the reduction in troop size due to the plague, all of these measures were necessary and sensible. However, if you were a man who had spent the last twenty years of your life fighting in the most glorious military in the world, and you noticed that your dead comrades had been replaced by octogenarian former slaves and horse thieves, you might get a sense that the place the army occupied in the Roman world had changed dramatically.

Economic problems also loomed. The plague meant that expenses for the military kept increasing; some units required two times as many recruits as they had in the past. Meanwhile, the plague also caused significantly less governmental income to come in from estates, because if your populace is crippled by disease no one's number one priority is making sure that their vineyards are superprofitable. The empire was forced into debt.

Marcus Aurelius, in a surprising move, began selling off his imperial property in the Forum of Trajan. According to the fourth-century historian Eutropius, the emperor

> held an auction in the Forum of the Deified Trajan of imperial furnishings, and sold gold, crystal, and myrrhine drinking vessels, even royal vases, his wife's silk and gold-embroidered clothing, even certain jewels . . . the sale went on for two months and such a quantity of gold was acquired

that after he had carried through the remainder of the Marcomannic war in accordance with his intentions, he gave
permission to buyers to return their purchases and get their
money back, if they wanted. He did not cause trouble to anyone, whether he returned what he had bought or not.[15]

I can't quite believe a ruler financed a war by having a crazy yard
sale, but ancient Rome is surprising in many ways.

At least temporarily, the auction worked. Marcus Aurelius
formed a new defensive zone, the Praetentura Italiae et Alpium, to
respond to the crisis on the border. There were setbacks—like the
killing of twenty thousand Roman troops by the Marcomanni
and their leader, Ballomar, near Carnuntum in 170—but by
172 the Marcomanni tribe was vanquished. A peace treaty was
signed with the remaining warring tribes (the Quadi and Sarma-
tians) in 175, whereupon the tribes agreed to release approximately 160,000 captured
Romans.[16] (I am end-noting
the preceding sentence as
much for my own benefit as
yours, because the number
is so large that I keep going
back to make sure I read it
correctly.)

Rome was ultimately
victorious in the wars against
the Marcomanni. If you
visit the column of Marcus
Aurelius—and you have
either a towering ladder or
excellent binoculars—you
can see carvings of the barbarian princes surrender-
ing to the emperor.

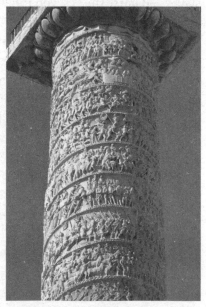

*A column was the highest honor available
at the time.*

So the Romans won in the end. But the Germanic tribes, by capturing hundreds of thousands of Romans and crossing the Danube, had dealt a decisive blow to any notion of Roman invulnerability, which was vital to the people of ancient Rome. I am going to quote from the television show *The West Wing* (1999–2006) here. It was historically accurate when President Josiah Bartlet said: "Two thousand years ago a Roman citizen could walk across the face of the known world free of the fear of molestation. He could walk across the Earth unharmed, cloaked only in the protection of the words civis romanus [sum] 'I am a Roman citizen.' So great was the retribution of Rome, universally understood as certain should any harm befall even one of its citizens." Lest you reply, "That is not historically accurate, Jennifer. That is *The West Wing*'s brilliant but erratic screenwriter Aaron Sorkin writing whatever he wants, and you just like it when President Bartlet says stuff like that." The Roman lawyer Cicero himself speaks of this sense of entitlement about two hundred years before the fall of Aquileia. When indicting a warlord named Verres for torturing a Roman citizen, Cicero writes:

No groan was heard, no expression was heard from that wretched man, amid all his pain, and between the sound of the blows except these words, "I am a citizen of Rome." He fancied that by this one statement of his citizenship he could ward off all blows . . . and you, Verres, you confess that he did cry out he was a Roman citizen . . . you suspected he was a spy. I do not ask what were your grounds for that suspicion. I impeach you by your own words. He said that he was a Roman citizen.[17]

There were nightmarish aspects to Roman society. Romans killed one another *all the time*. Shit flowed through their streets. But no empire has ever rivaled Rome for making its people believe that as long as they were Roman citizens, they were, to the extent one could be in a dangerous world, safe. How, after the siege of Aquileia, could any Roman citizen truly believe that again? About 160,000 Romans had been captured. Their borders had been breached. Their army would never be the same again. It wouldn't even look the same: the Marcomannic Wars would be the last time the lorica segmentata and rectangular shields would be used by the legionnaires. According to McLynn, "The legions lost both their clear social status and their clearly differentiated appearance."[18]

If Marcus Aurelius had lived longer, the empire might have recovered, if not its population, at least the sense of what it meant to be a Roman citizen. The nineteenth-century historian Barthold Georg Niebuhr wrote, "There can be no doubt that, during the last years of the war, the Romans were victorious, though not without the most extraordinary exertions, and that if M. Aurelius had lived longer, he would have made Marcomannia and Sarmatia Roman provinces."[19] That last part is speculative, but, sure! Maybe! Sensible rulers like Marcus Aurelius are without doubt a godsend in times of plague. Rome was fortunate to be led by a man who was able to respond calmly to each crisis with a rational—if sometimes unexpected—solution. People speak often about Marcus Aurelius's philosophical genius, his sense of morality, and his all-around greatness, and I'm sure all of that is true, but on a practical level the man was just an excellent problem solver. Like Matt Damon's character in *The Martian* (2015) good. During crises like the Antonine plague, being a problem solver is the best thing you can be. When we are electing government officials, it is not stupid to ask yourself, "If a plague broke out, do I think this person could navigate the country through those times, on a spiritual level, but also on a pragmatic one? Would they be able to calmly solve one problem, and then another one, and then the next one? Or would bodies pile up in the streets?" Certainly, it would be better than asking yourself if you would enjoy drinking a beer with them.

Unfortunately, despite Niebuhr's hopeful speculation, Marcus Aurelius *didn't* live longer. He died in 180, most likely of the plague. While he continued to believe that immorality was a greater evil than any disease, the plague was certainly on his mind. Supposedly his last words were, "Weep not for me; think rather of the pestilence and the deaths of so many others."[20] Gibbon claimed, "The ancient world never recovered from the blow inflicted on it by the plague which visited it in the reign of M. Aurelius."[21]

Gibbon got it right. Whether you attribute the beginning of the fall of Rome to the weakening of its military, the increased confidence and aggression of people outside its borders, the Romans' damaged national psyche, economic issues, or the untimely death of Marcus Aurelius—every one of those things was tied or directly attributable to the plague. The first lesson of this book is that plagues don't just affect a population's health. If they are not quickly defeated by medicine, any significant outbreak of disease sends horrible ripples through every aspect of society.

In the wake of the Antonine plague, Rome began a dizzying downward spiral.

The empire was not going to recover under the reign of Commodus, Marcus Aurelius's nineteen-year-old successor. Steering a civilization while a plague is constantly undermining it is like trying to captain a boat with a hole in its hull. Not only do you need to be able to pilot, you also have to devote an ungodly amount of time and effort to triaging the compounding emergencies. And even in the best of times, Commodus couldn't have captained a paddle boat across a kiddie pool. Dio writes that, when dealing with the Marcomanni immediately following Marcus Aurelius's death: "Commodus might easily have destroyed them, yet he made terms with them; for he hated all exertion and craved the comfortable life of the city."[22] Commodus is played by Joaquin Phoenix in *Gladiator* as a man whose defining trait is his desire to have sex with his sister, Lucilla. (That's debatable—he more likely had sex with his other sisters, not the one in the film.) My real quibble with the movie is that it left out so many more of Commodus's horrible traits. Dio claimed he was "not naturally wicked, but . . . [his] great simplicity, however, together with his cowardice, made him the slave of his companions . . . [by whom] he was led into lustful and cruel habits, which soon became second nature."[23] He frittered away his time as emperor in increasingly bizarre ways, such as, according to Dio, randomly changing his name to "Lucius Aelius Aurelius Commodus Augustus Herculeus Romanus Exsuperatorius Amazonius Invictus Felix Pius" and then demanding that the names of months on the calendar be changed to correspond with his made-up name. Maybe you think, *He was like the artist formerly known as Prince!* No. Prince changed his name because of a contract dispute. Commodus changed his name because his brain was full of dumb ideas and positive reinforcement. He spent the rest of his time poisoning his perceived political enemies and killing extremely unthreatening animals in gladiatorial games. Dio recalls an incident where he killed an ostrich and paraded it proudly before the senators, who had to restrain their laughter.

While Commodus was being a cowardly, banana-brained, ultimately assassinated monster, the Antonine plague segued into the Cyprian plague and didn't really end until 270. And, unlike during Marcus Aurelius's reign, rulers weren't constantly working to solve the myriad of issues a plague produces. By the time 270 rolled around, the emperor Valerian had already been captured and held hostage by the Persians, so that notion about the citizens of Rome being safe had flown way out the window. Barbarian tribes had become more aggressive; and while some integrated into Roman society, the far-flung portions of the empire began to break away. By 410 the city of Rome— Rome itself! Once home to over a million people during Marcus

Aurelius's reign!—would be sacked by Visigoths. The city was sacked *again* by Vandals in 440 and then *again* by the Ostrogoths in 547. By the time the Ostrogoths left, there were only a few hundred people left in the city. Thus the curtain rose on the Dark Ages, now euphemistically called the "Early Middle Ages" (which seems a lot like calling a mass unmarked grave an "early flower garden").

If someone were to exclaim, "I am a citizen of Rome!" today, it would not so much as gain a reprieve from a traffic ticket.

The takeaway from this story is that there is really only one thing we should collectively fear ending civilizations. It's not licentious behavior. If the biggest problem in your civilization is people having sex, you are doing great. It isn't even necessarily other countries attacking you because they hate you and all that you stand for. If you've got a big enough army you can fight them off. The real terror is plague. It's waiting out there, somewhere, under the ice or in a jungle. If it strikes and it can't be combatted effectively, it can take down an empire.

Bubonic Plague

*"I guess I'm the Black Death," he
said slowly. "I don't seem to bring
people happiness anymore."*

—*Tender Is the Night*, F. SCOTT FITZGERALD

One social media trick that makes me furious is when I encounter little pop-up ads saying that some doctor has found the cure for Alzheimer's disease. These messages enrage me because I know I'm going to click on them. I can't help it. I respond because I am absolutely terrified of getting Alzheimer's. I will click on those ads *every single time.*

Generally, the link takes you to a very long video of a man saying he has studied Alzheimer's for years and now you should buy his book. Which I'm not going to buy because there is currently no cure for Alzheimer's; if there were, it would be widely reported in the press, so that man would not have to make a homemade video to share his "cure." But . . . I am sure that if I clicked one of those messages and it just read in bold font, unsupported by any medical expertise, **Eat More Bananas,** I would eat more bananas.

I would do that even though I am a person of the twenty-first century who knows that you should look for some reliable proof of a treatment's effectiveness before you start any regimen. People—even fairly sane ones—seem to have an irrational tendency to respond to a fearsome disease by latching on to any supposed "cures" without proof of whether or not they would actually be helpful. It is hard to "keep calm and carry on" when you are scared.

This may explain why, when the bubonic plague began spreading through Europe in 1347, the average medieval person latched on to treatments that were absolutely, utterly insane.

During the fourteenth century, when the bubonic plague was at its most destructive, 90 percent of western Europeans were living off the land, mostly as farmers. There was a very small class of intelligentsia (who were probably dismissed as "not the REAL western Europeans"). If you were a peasant and someone said, "If you live in a sewer, the bubonic plague won't kill you," your reaction likely wouldn't be, "I am curious to hear the science behind that." Your response would be, "Point me to the nearest sewer." Terror over the devastating disease and a lack of scientific knowledge, as well as some people's truly evil tendency to prey upon people's fears, resulted in safeguards that seem ludicrous today.

In no particular order, these were some fourteenth-century methods thought to be effective against the bubonic plague:

DRINKING A SMALL AMOUNT OF GOOD WINE.

Fourteenth-century chronicler Gilles Li Muisis claimed that no one who drank wine in Tournai died. Sure! This is a great cure, actually. This one is valid for everything from minor colds to terminal illnesses. Or, if it's not (it is not), it at least seems to be fun. I wanted to begin with a cure that is fun.[1]

LIVING INSIDE A SEWER.

The reasoning behind this lifestyle choice seemed to be that your body would become so accustomed to filth and untold horrors that the plague could not harm it. This was wrong, especially as the plague is thought to have been carried by fleas on rats, many of which made their homes in sewers. So you'd be more likely to contract the plague, and you'd be living in a really awful place during your final days.[2]

EATING CRUSHED EMERALDS.

Yes, this behavior seems cool. It sounds like something a rich man in Greek mythology would do. But it is not a good idea at all. Emeralds have no value outside of humans' perception of their worth. They are just rocks. People were voluntarily swallowing shards of rocky glass, which had the potential to kill them by ripping their gastrointestinal tract and causing internal bleeding. Unless of course the emeralds were ground very, very finely—in which case there would be no effect whatsoever. (Fun fact: you can't kill someone by finely grinding up glass and mixing it in their food. Either they'd be able to detect it, or it would be too finely ground to kill them. I'm too smart for you, potential murderers who are after my history-book-writing fortune.)[3]

EATING EGGS, FRUITS, AND VEGETABLES.

Do we see a glimmer of the modern world? Eating these foods seems like common sense because they are packed with nutrients! But, no, that had nothing to do with that reasoning. Instead the advice had to do with avoiding foods like milk, cheese, and meat, or anything that would smell bad if it was left out in the sun. That's because it was believed that bad smells caused the plague. This notion, known as the miasma theory, regarding bad air, would persist, irritatingly, into the nineteenth century. People kind of lucked into this healthy eating regimen.[4]

NOT LOOKING AT SICK PEOPLE.

One doctor believed that "an aerial spirit" could fly out of a sick person's eyes and into another person's body, especially if you looked at that sick person while they were dying. This is not true, but I suppose you could avoid looking at anyone ever, just in case, as certain rock stars do.[5]

CHOPPING UP RAW ONIONS AND PLACING THEM THROUGHOUT YOUR HOUSE.

Since many people thought that the plague was spread through bad smells, they hoped that placing onions around the house would purify the air. It didn't. But the myth about chopped-up onions having healing properties became shocking prevalent. Even today the National Onion Association has to explain in its Frequently Asked Questions that placing chopped onions around your house will not prevent diseases. It is so strange and, I guess, quite selfless of the organization to do that. We should buy lots of onions to reward it for being honest. Sometimes, bubonic plague sufferers were given onion broth to drink. That was both because fourteenth-century people vastly overestimated onions' healing properties and because—as I learned from the National Onion Association—it is delicious and contains "layers of flavor."[6]

DRINKING YOUR URINE/BUBOES PUS.

In an attempt to expose their bodies to the disease and make them hardier, some people would drink pus from burst boils or their own urine (twice a day!). Needless to say, this tactic did not work, and it makes drinking onion broth or wine sound truly delightful in comparison.[7]

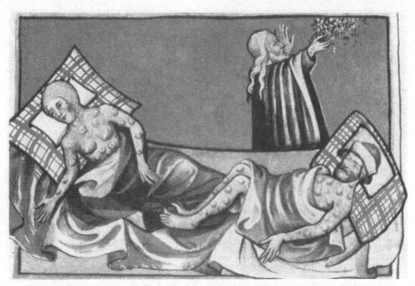

These guys were lucky—they had pillows and an in-home wizard.

For those of you who, having heard of these "cures," are curious about the real science of this plague, it is generally spread by flea bites. Certain rats carry—and can live with—a bacterium called *Yersinia pestis.* Fleas also live on rats, and when they suck rats' blood, they absorb that bacterium, which then multiplies in those fleas' stomachs. Then the rats carry the fleas to areas populated by humans. When a rat dies, the fleas jump to a new host, like a human. They bite the human host and leave traces of the bacteria in the wound. Some hosts then scratch or rub that area, driving the bacteria farther into the wound (though, honestly, not scratching doesn't seem to make much difference). The bacteria then make their way through the lymphatic system. This results in buboes, which appear on the body like boils. Hence the name "bubonic plague," although at the time the disease was more often referred to as "the Great Mortality" or, in France, "Le charbon," meaning coal or carbon, likely because of the buboes' lumpy, coal-like appearance. (And yes, the word *boo-boo* is thought to possibly be derived from *buboes*. You should never kiss a bubo to make it better.) The disease would come to be known as the Black Death.

Buboes are swollen lymph nodes, which usually develop in the armpits, genitals, or neck. So this disease began rather revoltingly with a golf ball–sized goiter under your armpit or in your groin. Jeuan Gethin, a Welshman living in 1349, recorded: "Woe is me of the shilling in the arm-pit; it is seething, terrible, wherever it may come . . . It is of the form of an apple, like the head of an onion, a small boil that spares no-one. Great is its seething, like a burning cinder, a grievous thing of an ashy colour."[8]

Here is an unsurprising fact: Gethin died of the bubonic plague almost immediately after writing this. Most people died within four days of exhibiting the first symptoms, and many died within twenty-four hours. The fourteenth-century author Boccaccio also writes about the same buboes Gethen describes, saying, "some waxed to the bigness of a common apple, others to the size of an egg."[9]

In addition to egg-sized buboes that oozed pus and blood, victims of the plague could expect a fever, vomiting, muscle aches, and delirium. There would also be subcutaneous hemorrhaging. That's because the bubonic plague inhibits the body's ability to clot blood. According to Boccaccio, this would result in "purple spots in most parts of the body: in some cases large and but few in number, in others less and more numerous, both sorts the usual messengers of death."[10] If the plague spread to the lungs and became pneumonic, it could be transmitted from person to person through an infected cough. The plague would kill somewhere between 20 and 50 million people in the fourteenth century, or approximately 30 percent of Europe's population.

Given the level of fear induced by this plague, the "eat more bananas/emeralds" prevention steps don't seem all that unreasonable. The more extreme steps to purportedly avoid the plague were based in religious fervor. It's not surprising that when a massive plague is killing even the wealthy emerald eaters, people turn to God. Many carved crosses on their doors in the hopes that the sign would cause the plague to pass by. That generally seems pretty harmless!

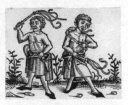

Seems like they had cool shoes, though.

But fourteenth-century life quickly became weirder. Many hoped that by flagellating themselves they might earn God's pardon. Largely from Holland, the flagellants spread through Europe during the mid-fourteenth century. They marched naked through cities, whipping themselves until they bled. They also weren't allowed to wash their wounds or talk to women. They would fling themselves facedown with their arms spread out like the cross. They would do this over and over, for thirty-three and a third days in each place they visited. The number of days was supposed to represent the number of years Christ lived on earth. Pope Clement VI officially forbade the activity in October 1349, but by then, zealots had largely turned their attention from hurting themselves to harming the Jews. The widespread rumor was that the Jews were going around dumping the plague into wells. Seemingly, medieval Christians remembered essentially nothing from the horrors of their own persecution in Rome because they did not hesitate to form large mobs and attack Jews.

Pope Clement attempted to stem this outbreak of anti-Semitism by issuing a bull saying that anyone who thought the Jews were actually responsible for the plague "had been seduced by that liar, the devil,"[11] and that the killings should stop. That was a wonderful move. Pope Clement's well-intentioned bull was said to calm tensions in some regions, like France and Italy, but other parts of Europe weren't as receptive. If you do a quick Google search on this topic, you will find that some hateful people still believe—today!—that the bubonic plague was deliberately spread by Jews poisoning wells. That rumor, though medically implausible, is apparently sufficiently compelling to continue to appeal to poorly informed people. So it is horrifying but not wholly unexpected that in February 1349, nine hundred Jews were burned to death in Strasbourg. A chronicler wrote: "They were led to their own cemetery into a house prepared for their burning and on their way were stripped naked by the crowd which ripped off their clothes."[12] In the same year, in Mainz, six thousand Jews were supposed to have been killed on a single day, and over twenty thousand were murdered in total.

King Casimir of Poland, who had a Jewish mistress, offered refuge in his country to all Jews seeking to escape persecution.

So, nice job, King Casimir. I hope you receive a History Channel special.

But it wasn't only religious zealots who were causing mayhem. In Italy a group of gravediggers with the motto "Those who live in fear die" were especially menacing. They were called the *becchini*, and, though this is not historically accurate, in my head they look exactly like the gang of droogs in the movie *A Clockwork Orange* (1971). John Kelly writes: "The terrors of life in Florence grew to include a front door bursting open in the dead of night and a group of drunken, shovel-wielding grave diggers rushing into the house, threatening rape and murder unless the inhabitants paid a ransom."[13] Periodically, they threatened to drag people who were still alive to the grave if they weren't paid. As if there weren't enough dead people around.

Societal order was breaking down in every respect. Cities that had once been lovely were becoming mass graves. Boccaccio writes that plague pits of the deceased were so full in Florence that the dead had to be "stored tier upon tier like ship's cargo, each layer of corpses being covered with a thin layer of soil til the trench was fill to the top."[14] The Florentine Marchionne di Coppo Stefani said that the pits looked like lasagna.[15] (This image may ruin the Olive Garden for you forever.) But Florence had a slightly better corpse situation than Siena, of which the chronicler Agnolo di Tura writes, "There were also those who were so sparsely covered with earth that the dogs dragged them forth and devoured many bodies throughout the city."[16] This is what happens when a society does not have Marcus Aurelius to keep the bodies out of the streets.

All of these details can blur together a bit, so take a minute to consider what it would be like to see wild dogs dragging around human remains in front of your house. Then consider gravediggers running through town screaming, "Those who live in fear die," while threatening to rape you. (For the purposes of this exercise, the *becchini* aren't discriminating based on gender.) Then overlay the religious zealots parading their bloodied bodies on the streets, and the stench of burned Jewish corpses in the air, and I think you will have a good sense of how awful it would be to live in the time of the bubonic plague.

Now maybe eat a cupcake and take a bath; you earned it.

No one wanted to live in this hellscape. Everyone who could escape the lasagna-plague-pit-filled cities fled. Boccaccio's novel *The Decameron*, which takes place in 1349, begins with a group of aristocrats bolting to the country to escape the plague. They do so not only "to preserve their lives" from the plague but to protect themselves from those given over to bestial behavior. Early in the novel the aristocrats came to an agreement:

> [We should] make our retreate to our Country houses, wherewith all of us are sufficiently furnished, and there to delight our selves as best we may, yet without transgressing (in any act) the limits of reason. There shall we heare the pretty birds sweetly singing, see the hilles and plaines verdantly flouring; the Corne waving in the field like the billowes of the Sea, infinite store of goodly trees, and the Heavens more fairely open to us, then here we can behold them . . . Moreover, the Ayre is much fresh and cleere, and

generally, there is farre greater abundance of all things whatsoever, needefull at this time for preservation of our health,
and lesse offence or mollestation then we find here.[17]

Not everyone had a country house, so most people had to be
content with leaving their immediate surroundings in favor of
any place that seemed marginally less deadly. There are stories
about how common it was for people to leave bread and water at
a sick relative's bedside, tell them they were going out to fetch
supplies, and then abandoning them. The dying could be seen
through the city plaintively rapping at their windows, hoping
someone would come to ease their suffering. The fourteenth-
century historian Gabriel de Mussis remarks upon how, as
people died, they still begged for their families to come to them:
"Come here, I'm thirsty, bring me a drink of water. I'm still
alive. Don't be frightened. Perhaps I won't die. Please hold me
tight, hug my wasted body. You ought to be holding me in your
arms."[18] De Mussis describes the streets ringing with the cries
of dying children who had been locked out of their homes, and
who wondered: "Father, why have you abandoned me? Do you
forget I am your child? O, Mother, where have you gone? Why
are you now so cruel to me when yesterday you were so kind?
You fed me at your breast and carried me within your womb for
nine months."[19]

If upon reading of these heartrending cries, you are thinking that you would be a heroic time traveler, rushing to those
dying people's aid, then let me stop you right there. First, your
decision to travel to the plague-ridden fourteenth century is
exceedingly ill-advised. I can only assume that in this fantasy
you are a reporter for the *Vice* TV series. Second, no one wanted
to force their children into the streets. No one wanted to leave
them to die alone. They did so only because doing otherwise
would doom them also. You could go to those children, but you
would almost certainly die, because if the disease had spread to

the victims' lungs, they were contagious and could spread the disease by coughing on you. People were put in the nightmarish position where they could die alongside their loved ones or live and allow their loved ones to die utterly alone.

John Kelly explains the psychology of plague times in modern-day terms: "In plague, fear acts as a solvent on human relationships; it makes everyone an enemy and everyone an isolate. In plague every man becomes an island—a small, haunted island of suspicion, fear, and despair."[20] The fourteenth-century chronicler Agnolo di Tura summed up the age when he wrote: "Father abandoned child, wife husband, one brother another; for this illness seemed to strike through breath and sight. And so they died. None could be found to bury the dead for money or friendship. I, Agnolo di Tura ... buried my five children with my own hands ... And so many died that all believed it was the end of the world."[21]

The Italian poet and humanist Petrarch certainly had every reason to believe the world was ending. He lost his great love Laura to the plague in 1348. Meanwhile, his brother was in a monastery where the other thirty-five inhabitants had died, leaving him alone with only his dog for company. Just him, his dog, and thirty-five corpses. Petrarch wrote to him, "I would, my brother, that I had never been born, or, at least, had died before these times ... O happy posterity, who will not experience such abysmal woe and will look upon our testimony as a fable."[22]

I worry, sometimes, that we do look on this plague as a far-removed fable, without remembering the very real cries of those on their deathbeds begging to be hugged.

In spite of the fear and isolation the plague produced, there were still doctors who attempted to minister to the sufferers. Some of the plague doctors were altruists who wanted to help their dying countrymen. Others were second-rate physicians who saw treating plague patients as their only way to make a living in medicine. That was especially true as plague doctors became so essential they were often employed by towns rather than individuals. They were outfitted with massive waxed robes and a staff to indicate their profession. They also—and this is where the term *beak doctor* comes in—wore bird-shaped masks.

Now, there is some conflict as to when this garb was introduced. While the majority of this chapter focuses on the bubonic plague's impact on fourteenth- to sixteenth-century Europe, the plague continued to rage through Europe until the eighteenth century. It's possible this type of outfit wasn't worn until the seventeenth century. However, some sources attribute its origins to the fourteenth. I think it's worth describing regardless of when it was introduced, but for you time travelers, do not bank on this outfit being available before 1619.

Although people at the time didn't exactly know why, the beak doctor's outfits did, miraculously, offer protection. You might not immediately guess that, as some of the logic behind their construction was bizarre. For instance, the mask was shaped like a bird because people thought birds could frighten away plague demons. People must have really liked birds back then.

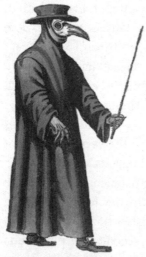

Like Big Bird, but slightly less creepy

The beaks of those bird masks were stuffed with anything that smelled good. That could be a veritable potpourri from mint to rose petals to orange peels. The sweet-scented items were thought to prevent the doctors from breathing the poisonous air. Remember that people believed bad smells caused plagues. The glass eyes fitted onto the masks would supposedly stop doctors from contracting the plague via the evil eye, preventing the "aerial spirits" from reaching them.

This all sounds like superstitious nonsense, but each aspect of the costume also served a purpose modern people would recognize as practical. The long, black waxed robes that went to the ground ensured that the doctors were bitten by very few fleas and thus were less likely to contract the disease through its most common source. The masks—with their glass eyes—provided distance between them and any cough droplets their patients might be spewing. The fact that it smelled like a Bath and Body Works store inside the masks meant the doctors were less disgusted by the smells of death and decay in a sufferer's house and thus willing to spend more time with their patients. The staffs— well, they used their staffs to beat patients sometimes. For real! They did that when patients lunged at them, which is not very doctor-y but is helpful to keep infected people at a distance. Hopefully more often, though, a doctor would use the staff to point to areas of the body without actually touching the patient.

If only the "medical" methods of treating the disease had been anywhere near as effective as the outfit. If you were being tended to by a bubonic plague doctor in the fourteenth century, you could expect:

THE EXPLODING-FROG CURE.

People have been terrified of frogs through much of history. Today, the notion of a princess kissing a frog seems cute and funny, but historically, that would have been the most repellent act imaginable. Part of the bias against frogs might be because they were associated with this cure. The "exploding frog cure" was almost certainly not its technical name. It's definitely the only way I'll ever refer to it, though. Plague doctors would place a frog belly down on one of the patient's buboes. The frog would absorb the poison, swell up, and ultimately explode. Then they'd do it with another frog, and another, until the frogs stopped exploding. If a frog did not explode, that meant the patient would die. This may be the most insane, ineffective cure in the world, but if you have the opportunity to travel back in time, *please* go see it performed, even though visiting the fourteenth century is dumb, so dumb, just so dumb.[23]

THE PIGEON CURE.

This is similar to the frog cure except the pigeons didn't explode; they just died. The method dictated that doctors should "take a Pigeon, and plucke the feathers off her taile, very bare, and set her taile to the sore, and shee will draw out the venome till shee die; then take another and set too likewise, continuing so till all the venome be drawne out, which you shall see by the Pigeons, for they will die with the venome as long as there is any in it: also chicken or a henne is very good."[24] From that addendum about how chickens and hens would work in a pinch, I have the sense that people were just randomly applying any household creature they could catch to the afflicted's wounds.

THE FIG AND ONION CURE.

Onions continued to be a real medicinal staple during this period. When people weren't spreading them around the house, figs and onions and butter would be applied to the sores to soften them. After some time, the buboes would be cut into so the poison could drain out. You were to: "take a greate onion, hollow it, put into it a fig cut small and a dram of Venice treacle, put it close stopt in wet paper and roast it in the embers, apply it hot unto the tumour."[25] You were supposed to apply a boiling onion to your sore. This method was, as you might imagine, as painful as it was useless.

BLOODLETTING AND FECES POULTICES.

Sometimes (not often) the boils burst, and then the patient recovered. But covering the burst buboes with poultices that contained, among other things, feces, was a step back in the recovery journey. I realize that "Do No Harm" is the first rule of medicine, but "Don't apply human shit to an open wound" seems like a good second one. Oh, and bloodletting didn't help, either.[26]

‡—

Obviously, the first priority in combatting plague should be creating an environment where there are fewer rats harboring fleas. This has nothing to do with flagellating yourself or collecting frogs.

The first person who combatted the bubonic plague in any sort of sensible or helpful way was Michel de Nostredame, more familiarly known as Nostradamus. Born in 1503, Nostradamus is sometimes reported to be a wizard who predicted the end of the world. People have come to think he had magical abilities because Nostradamus spent his later years sitting in a castle with his wealthy second wife, writing books of predictions about events he thought would happen. Those publications were common for somewhat famous people to produce at the time. Our equivalent might be if Warren Buffett wrote a book about where he thinks the economy will be in the future. That's not the same as being a wizard. That's just a thing people who are famous for being smart do.

I am only eager to dispel the notion that Nostradamus was an otherworldly wizard because I think it overshadows the fact that he was a learned and progressive man, and those skills are as valuable as wizardry. They're also skills humans can actually cultivate. His powers didn't come from the heavens; they came from the fact that he was an avid reader, interested in the

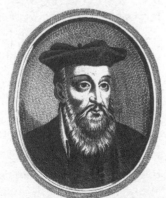

Not a real wizard despite the beard

scientific advances of his own time, as well as the medical arts of the past. As a teenager, he was seen as something of an oddball because he was convinced that the earth revolved around the sun in the manner Copernicus described, an idea which went against the church's view. (He was right about that.) However, more relevant to his work with the ill and his ideas about how to treat plague outbreaks was likely Nostradamus's admiration for the writings of Galen. In 1558 he would even publish his own translation of Menodotus's paraphrase of Galen.

Long before that, though, he spent the 1520s working as an apothecary preparing pills, and starting a doctorate at the University of Montpellier. There is a disputed rumor that he was expelled from the school because he had worked in an apothecary, which wasn't seen as a respectable practice. Many people just ground up anything and sold their "magic" medications, but Nostradamus's pills kind of worked. (We'll get to them later in this chapter, but they were essentially vitamin C.) He went back to his trade through the 1530s, becoming especially intent on helping treat the bubonic plague.

It has been reported that Nostradamus began contemplating treatments for the bubonic plague when he saw a sufferer waving to him from her window. Again, this was not an uncommon sight. When he went closer to her window, he saw that she was so certain of her imminent death that she had already begun stitching her shroud around herself. By the time Nostradamus entered her house, the woman had died "with her shroud half sewn."[27] That is such a good anecdote! Though surely at least part of his motivation to deal with the plague had to be that his first wife and two daughters died from the disease in the 1530s.

Without antibiotics no one could truly cure people once they had the plague, but Nostradamus was unusually successful at finding effective methods to deter the disease. Many of those methods stemmed from Nostradamus's own rather modern preferences regarding cleanliness (which might have been influenced from his reading of classic texts, like Galen's). Some of Nostradamus's methods included:

GETTING THE CORPSES OUT OF THE STREET.

Obviously, having corpse pits is a disaster. You need to bury the dead if only because having them lying around is a surefire way to attract those flea-carrying rats. Also, when people see bodies lying in the streets, they become absolutely terrified. Given that fear is the enemy of reason during disease outbreaks, it's a good idea to try to keep those streets clean.[28]

REMOVING SOILED LINENS.

Nostradamus wasn't the first person to decide that sheets or clothing people have died in shouldn't be kept around. Galen was also keen on the idea that people ought to clean their clothes. Closer to Nostradamus's own time, Boccaccio writes of an incident where "the rags of a poor man just dead, being thrown into the street, and two hogs coming by at the same time and rooting amongst them, and shaking them about in their mouths, in less than an hour turned round and died on the spot."[29] Filthy bedding provided an especially great home to plague-carrying fleas. Disposing of linens should be easy, but think about how much you hate the idea of changing your sheets when you're sick. Now think about a world where many people wore the same outfit for a whole year, and where no one had taught you that changing linens was a chore you were supposed to do. Still, society was making progress![30]

DRINKING BOILED WATER.

Though not as much fun as imbibing wine or onion broth, drinking boiled water was effective, especially when the rivers were swimming with corpses. Seriously, just *full* of corpses. The pope had to bless the Rhône River in France because it contained so many bodies and people wanted to believe their loved ones were in holy ground. Although the bubonic plague wasn't transmitted by water, drinking contaminated water could result in independent health problems, which could weaken a person's immune system and make them more susceptible to the plague.[31]

BATHING.

Good hygiene practices greatly reduce the risk of flea infestations. Nostradamus himself bathed daily. However, that was an anomaly. Most people in medieval times took two baths a year. Bathing was thought to cause disease and death by widening the pores and allowing the plague to enter the body more easily. Nostradamus may have developed this revolutionary bathing theory from his reading of history. Galen not only encouraged bathing but was the first doctor to recommend people clean themselves with soap.[32]

GETTING FRESH AIR.

Many people shut themselves up in sick rooms. Even more so when people were afraid that the air itself was polluted with plague. Pope Clement VI famously surrounded himself with torches to try to burn away the supposedly poisonous fumes. Going outside and getting exercise, especially in the countryside, could be effective in boosting the immune system. The 10 percent of those who recovered from the plague generally had robust and healthy immune systems.[33]

EATING A MAGIC PILL.

Many people on the Internet want to credit Nostradamus's success in combatting the plague to the fact that he had a magic wizard pill. He didn't. But he did make a "rose pill" that was a good source of vitamin C. People were making pills with absolutely everything in them—that's why being an apothecary wasn't seen as a respectable practice—so it seems like kind of a fluke that this pill worked when so many others failed. But, yes, taking vitamin C every day, especially if your diet is otherwise lacking in it, generally strengthens immune systems. Would you like to know the recipe for the magic pill? I would, because I like those books where, say, Nora Ephron gives me a fun recipe halfway through a chapter. This is probably as close as I'm ever going to get to being able to do that:

RECIPE

Take some sawdust or shavings of cypress-wood, as green as you can find, one ounce; iris of Florence, six ounces; cloves, three ounces; sweet calamus [cane palm], three drams; aloes-wood six drams. Grind everything to powder and take care to keep it all airtight. Next, take some furled red roses, three or four hundred, clean, fresh, and culled before dewfall. Crush them to powder in a marble mortar, using a wooden pestle. Then add some half-unfurled roses to the above powder and pound. And shape into pills.[34]

I look forward to seeing some intrepid twenty-first-century florist make and market this magic pill. It has a pretty good track record! In Aix-en-Provence, according to lore, Nostradamus's remedies spared the entire town from the plague. The town rewarded him with a lifelong stipend. He was, shortly after, summoned to treat similar outbreaks in Lyon and Salon-de-Provence, where he remained until the end of his life.

Fairy-tale summary: everyone followed Nostradamus's advice, and the bubonic plague went away forever.

Unfortunately, not quite. Nostradamus himself was skeptical as to whether his advice ever proved as wondrous as the people in Aix-en-Provence thought it to be. A very good sign that someone is not a charlatan is that they are doubtful of their own skills and do not demand huge sums of money for a magical cure they say only they can provide. As to whether or not

Nostradamus's methods were utterly essential or only very mildly helpful, we can say, "Well, both." All of his ideas were so much better than stuffing live pigeons into sores. We could view "drinking clean water" and "not sleeping in soiled linens" as some of the first building blocks in what would become modern sanitation and public health. Basic hygiene and healthy practices in an age rife with misguided "cures" was true progress.

That said, even if you went for long walks and popped those vitamin C pills like M&M's, it would not necessarily stop you from getting the plague in the sixteenth century. It would make dying from it a little less likely, but if you got it, you would probably still die.

Still, by the eighteenth century, outbreaks of the bubonic plague had become much less common than during medieval times. That decrease was largely due to more societies developing basic standards of sanitation and to making improvements in personal hygiene. The streets of Germany, for instance, are no longer filled with garbage and feces, hygiene is standard, and there aren't many dead bodies lying around being tugged upon by dogs. All of this means a less hospitable environment for plague-carrying fleas.

But the bubonic plague never went away entirely. It still exists today. The World Health Organization reports that in 2013 there were 783 cases worldwide; 126 people died.[35] About ten people contract the disease in the United States every year. If you have been out hiking in a dry area like the American Southwest and find egg-shaped growths developing under your armpit, it is exceedingly important that you go to a doctor within twenty-four hours. Maybe it's a normal rash, but maybe you have the plague, so you should check that out really quickly, as quickly as you can. Fortunately, today the disease is generally treated with the antibiotic streptomycin and is curable so long as it is caught early.

The solutions Nostradamus proposed seem so obvious now, in this very clean world filled with antibiotics. "Don't sleep in filth. Bathe yourself." Yes. *Of course* those ideas are right. It's easy to scoff at anyone who thought exploding frogs like firecrackers was a good cure, especially when the cause of the disease seems so apparent now. There's even a great satirical article from the *Onion* titled "Rat-Shit-Covered Physicians Baffled by Spread of Black Plague," with excellent lines like: "surely some unknown, diseas'd element is to blame. Any fool can see that. It is as plain as the fleas in the feculent water we drink, of which there are so very, very many."[36]

But have some sympathy for the people gobbling down their emeralds. It is disheartening to think how simple and straight-forward the cures for the diseases that we are desperately researching today will seem to people in the future, when it will be known that *of course* you eat five bananas a day to prevent Alzheimer's.

One of the most heartbreaking accounts of the plague is that of the Florentine historian Giovanni Villani. Described by John Kelly as a generally blunt and somewhat crusty historian, Villani wrote an account of the plague with the final line, "The plague lasted until . . ."[37] The date was left blank because he died before the plague came to an end. He waited his whole life to fill in a date that never came.

Regardless of the age we're living in, many of us expect ill-nesses to be cured within our lifetimes. Sadly, that is not often the case.

Nevertheless, we can take some heart. Practically no one dies of bubonic plague now. It was one of the human race's most terrifying adversaries for many years, and we beat it, first with a bar of soap in the sixteenth century and then with antibiotics in the twentieth. Villani might hear that news and say, in a crotchety fashion, "Well, that's no good to me, I'm dead." Not everyone lives to see the end of a battle. I don't know if everyone battling the worst diseases we suffer today would feel comforted to know that one day humans will emerge victorious. All the same, I like to think about the ever-so-slightly smarter, saner people of the future looking back on our diseases and regarding them as they might a bizarre bunch of exploding frogs.

Dancing Plague

Time rushes by
love rushes by
life rushes by
but the
Red Shoes go on.

—*"The Red Shoes,"* LEONARD COHEN

Can human kindness and the support of your community cure disease? Not... generally. You will likely have better luck with antibiotics or vaccines. However, you only need to visit your local drugstore to see greeting cards and motivational posters (emblazoned with pictures of sunny fields, kittens, rainbows, and cartoon lambs) that have capitalized upon kindly sentiments where someone is sending "tender loving care for your recovery!" and "hugs to heal." I happened upon one that said, "I hope you get butter soon," accented with pictures of yellow sticks of butter.

These cards are lovely to receive, no doubt. Except for the butter one. That one is awful—unless you are giving it to someone with high cholesterol, in which case it is hilarious. However, if you suggested someone heal their cancer with hugs, they would rightly stare at you as if you had joined a murder cult.

Modern antibiotics, vaccinations, and drugs for life-threatening diseases have all of those saccharine wellness sayings at a distinct disadvantage. If you have to choose between living in an isolated, uncaring community with plentiful penicillin or a very warm and loving world without drugs, team up with the guys with penicillin. It's a lot easier to make people nicer than it is to develop medicine.

However, in the sixteenth century, those kindly sentiments were about all people had. And though they might not be as powerful as modern medicine, there is reason to believe that being treated with kindness and receiving the support of the community *do* help people recover from ailments. At least, they do if it is the sufferers' state of mind that is affecting their health. It's not as good as penicillin. But it's something. At least, it was in the case of the Dancing Plague.

The dancing plague started innocuously enough. In Strasbourg, in July 1518, a woman named Frau Troffea began dancing in the street.

To modern minds, the thought of anyone dancing probably conjures an image of someone who is happy or celebrating or listening to some cool music or, at the very least, drunk. That is a testament to the fact that we live in a world filled with music and causes for celebration. You could dance a jig in a supermarket if you wanted to. It would be weird, but people would just think you really, really liked Peter Gabriel and that there was a great sale on Pringles.

Not so in the sixteenth century, an age with less omnipresent music and virtually nothing to celebrate. The years surrounding 1518 were awful. This was a century of plagues, famine, and war. But none of that stopped people from dancing! They danced a lot but not because they were happy. They did so because they were nearly mad with woe. In *The Dancing Plague: The Strange,*

True Story of an Extraordinary Illness, the historian John Waller writes: "It was a world so glutted with misery that nearly all ranks of society drank and danced whenever the opportunity, with the intensity of those in flight from an intolerable reality."[1]

It was a truly terrible time to be alive in Alsace. I know throughout this book on plagues we won't encounter many good years, but this period was particularly dreadful. The year 1517 was so awful that it was sometimes simply called "the bad year."[2] Taxes had been at an all-time high, and crop yield was low, resulting in great famine made worse by the fact that peasants had been forbidden from fishing in streams and hunting in the local woods. Think *The Hunger Games* (book or movie), District 12. Smallpox ravaged Strasbourg while the bubonic plague broke out in Mulhouse. Many of the region's young men had been killed battling the Turks. The superstitious claimed they could see the dead roaming the streets at night. Dancing was a way to escape the nightmarish world through physical exertion, the way you might decide to hit the gym hard after a bad day at work. (Not because it's fun, just because it will take your mind off that monster, Charlie in Accounting.)

It was in this context that Frau Troffea began her dance.

A lone dancer in the middle of town would probably have initially been greeted with interest, if not surprise. While walking around the city, you might even respond to this nonthreatening but unexpected event with pleasure. (Full disclosure: I hate it—*hate* it—when the "showtime" guys dance on the Manhattan subway. But some people like that kind of thing, and I am trying to please all my readers.)

Sadly, as far as was recorded, Frau Troffea experienced absolutely no pleasure in her dance. And if people found it vaguely amusing at first, they seemed to find it odd by the end of the day. Some onlookers suspected that Frau Troffea was only carrying on because "nothing annoyed her husband more than just dancing."[3] People thought she was dancing wildly to perhaps make some kind of elaborate point to him. The physician Paracelsus suggested in his 1532 writings (I imagine while shaking his head at women and their horrible ways) that Frau Troffea kept dancing because her husband "told her to do something that she did not care for." He continued: "In order to make sure that her actions had their full effect and had the likeness of a disease, she hopped and jumped high, sang and lulled, and did whatever it was that her husband hated worst of all."[4] As if she were some sort of 1970s performance artist who wanted to make a point about being free to express her independent womanhood through movement.

Whenever there is an outbreak of mass hysteria, some people always decide the victims are faking it.

After some time, rather than going home to do sixteenth-century wifely duties, Frau Troffea passed out in the street. As Paracelsus put it: "After the completion of her dance, she collapsed in order to offend her husband. She jerked a while, and after that went to sleep. She claimed that all of this had been a disease attack, and said no more than this in order to make a fool of her husband."[5] As soon as she woke up, she started dancing again.

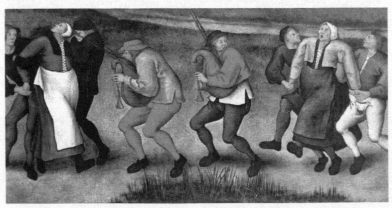

The Reverend in Footloose *was right: Dancing kills.*

By the third day blood was oozing out of her shoes, but still she danced. If she was merely doing this to annoy her husband, who admittedly sounds very uncool, she certainly would have stopped. By then, everyone was watching with horror rather than amusement. Soon dozens of other townspeople would mysteriously follow her lead.

Today, some sources claim that the root of this dancing plague lay with mold. Many outbreaks of the dancing plague (there were others!) happened near rivers where stalks of rye grew. Ergot is a kind of mold that can develop on those stalks. If you eat this ergot-infected rye, you can suffer horrible symptoms. The first among them might be a feeling of burning in your limbs. That burning is sometimes called "St. Anthony's Fire" because monks of the Antonine Order opened the Hospital of St. Anthony in 1075 to treat people suffering from ergot poisoning.

Ingesting ergot did cause people to convulse and experience hallucinations, but convulsing is not the same thing as dancing. If someone were onstage at the Grammys, you would be able to tell whether they were dancing or having a seizure, right? (Don't make a joke about how kids dance today; it will make you sound like Frau Troffea's husband.) And nowadays the rules for what constitutes dance are much less restrictive than they were five hundred years ago. In the sixteenth century learning various dances was considered a part of a young person's education. These dances were constructed with a mathematical precision that's different from what we think of when we consider dance today. None of them looked like convulsions. People at the time certainly would have known the difference and wouldn't say that someone spasming was dancing. And they are repeatedly clear that Frau Troffea and her followers were dancing. Besides, people were familiar with the symptoms of commonplace ergot poisoning. If Frau Troffea had it, she would have been taken to the Antonine brothers. The town dancers wouldn't have been considered to be suffering from a "strange epidemic"; they'd be suffering from a "normal epidemic."

All of this is to say that I really don't believe this plague was the work of a fungus. Nor did anyone at the time, though for less scholarly reasons.

The sixteenth-century layman's thinking about anyone developing a disorder was generally *God hates them because they're bad*. So by the standards of the time, most people would reason that Frau Troffea was being punished by God for something sinful. Paracelsus fell into that category. After deciding that the disease was real, Paracelsus claimed that "whores and scoundrels" were afflicted because their thoughts were "free, lewd and impertinent, full of lasciviousness and without fear or respect." He asserted that these depraved thoughts could come about by cursing too much or thinking about sex too much or the especially vague "corruption of the imagination."[6]

Those thoughts and acts could apply to many of us today. And yet most of us do not dance as though a bizarre curse has been placed upon us. However, Paracelsus wasn't *totally* off base when it comes to modern-day understanding of hysterical outbreaks. The modern Dr. Scott Mendelson writes about Freud's notion of "conversion disorder"—a condition in which you experience symptoms, like an inability to stop dancing, without any physical cause. When the condition spreads to other people, it is categorized as mass hysteria, or as it's often called today, mass psychogenic illness. "The disorder," explains Mendelson, "is thought to be driven by a subconscious attempt to 'convert' a strong, unbearable emotional or sexual thought into something more socially acceptable."[7] Experiencing conversion disorder doesn't necessarily mean that people go dancing in the streets uncontrollably. Symptoms can be much milder. For instance, when put in a stressful situation, women (or men) who have been socialized to suppress their anger might experience numbness in their hands or difficulty swallowing, or they might vomit.[8] This is your body saying, "Hey, shouldn't we be doing something now? Oh, we can't yell or punch people even though we're angry? We can't even think about being angry? Okay, we will do . . . something else. It's going to be weird!"

In the modern age, having sexual thoughts is generally socially acceptable. We don't need to suppress them so much we turn them into frantic dances. But life was different back then. Having sexual thoughts was a sure sign that not only were you going to hell, but you might deserve to be burned alive before you got there. In the fifteenth century the witch hunter's bible, the *Malleus Maleficarum*, claimed:

> If the world could be rid of women, we should not be without God in our intercourse . . . Witchcraft comes from carnal lust, which is in women insatiable. See Proverbs 30: There are three things that are never satisfied, yea, a fourth thing which says not "it is enough"; that is, the mouth of the womb. Wherefore for the sake of fulfilling their lusts they consort even with devils . . . witchcraft is high treason against God's Majesty. And so they are to be put to torture.[9]

The *Malleus Maleficarum* goes on to complain that while torture used to entail the accused being eaten by wild animals, now they're just being burned at the stake and that "probably this is because the majority of them are women."[10] Typical women. So entitled.

I cannot imagine a better reason to try to repress any sexual, lustful thoughts than knowing they would result in horrible torture. Whenever someone begins pompously complaining that civilization is on a downhill slide, because people participate in harmless behaviors like taking selfies or watching reality television, a good response is to stare at them and respond, "You know, we used to burn people for being witches. That's what people used to do in their spare time."

So Paracelsus might have been right in considering that the disease could have been caused by sexy thoughts. But only because people may have felt a desperate need to repress their "depravity" for fear of becoming devil worshippers.

Paracelsus was almost certainly wrong about how to *cure* the outbreak, however. He thought the best treatment, if the condition was brought on by cursing, was to have the dancers make an image of themselves in wax (talented multitasking dancers!), project their thoughts onto the wax doll, and then set the figure on fire. If the disease was brought on by sexy thoughts or frivolity, the dancers should be kept in a dark room and fed only bread and water until they were too sad to have those thoughts anymore. If it was caused by a "corrupt imagination," they should ingest opium (the basis for heroin) or alcohol.

Those were terrible guesses. They were bad tries. Maybe it was fortunate that his medical observations did not exist in 1518 when Frau Troffea began her dance, or she might well have attempted them.

As it was, the town generally decided that Frau Troffea was being punished by St. Vitus, the patron saint of dancers, who, I guess, just hated some people. In the sixteenth century it was common to curse someone by shouting, "God give you St. Vitus!"[11] As far back as the fourteenth century it was known that if you cursed someone that way, "the cursed person developed a fever and St. Vitus' dance."[12] I'm not saying you should curse people in the name of St. Vitus before they curse you, but I'm not *not* saying that.

Since the people believed St. Vitus had it out for Frau Troffea, they thought that if she worshipped before him she might be cured. She was, accordingly, driven off to his shrine in a wagon.

I know that I am setting low standards for human behavior here, but it is *astonishing* that the townspeople agreed they should try to help her rather than burn her as a witch. John

Waller notes, "Never were [the sufferers of the dancing plague] hauled before the inquisition,"[13] as they might have been if they were thought to be voluntary followers of Satan. That is shocking! The famous Würzburg and Bamberg witch trials in Germany, in which hundreds of people would be burned at the stake for less peculiar behavior, would happen less than a decade later. Go citizens of Strasbourg! You behaved significantly better than the norms of your century!

Was Frau Troffea cured? We have no information. We do know, however, that within a few days thirty people had followed her dancing lead, equally joylessly. Their feet bled until you could see their bones. *Their bones were poking through their flesh.* People kept dancing until they had heart attacks or collapsed from dehydration or infection (not surprising since their bones were sticking out of their feet). Waller explains: "They almost certainly were delirious. Only in an altered state of consciousness could they have tolerated such extreme fatigue and the searing pain of sore, swollen and bleeding feet. Moreover witnesses consistently spoke of the victims as being entranced, seeing terrifying visions and behaving with wild, crazy abandon."[14]

Remarkably, this behavior wasn't altogether uncommon. The outbreak of 1518 was not even the first instance of the dancing plague. There had been seven similar outbreaks in Europe since 1017. Frau Troffea's dance was just the first to be widely reported, likely because Strasbourg had a printing press. None of the prior epidemics gave people any clue how to handle the condition. For instance, although we are not absolutely sure this story is true, it was reported that during the outbreak of 1017, the local priest, who did not care for dancing, cursed everyone dancing to continue for an entire year. I am so infatuated with stories of religious officials going around cursing people as though that is a judicious use of power.

In 1247 about one hundred children danced out of the

German town of Erfurt, which sounds really cute until you take into account that by the time their parents found them, many were dead. In 1278 two hundred people danced, again, seemingly joylessly, over an unstable bridge, which collapsed, killing all of them. In 1347 dancers in the Rhineland "cried out, like lunatics, that they were dying."[15]

Let us be absolutely clear that no one was dancing because they wanted to dance, or because they were involved in some sort of cool cult that necessitated dancing. So it is sort of bizarre that Strasbourg initially responded as though everyone was doing this for fun.

Guildhalls in Strasbourg were opened to provide music as people danced, madly and miserably, to their deaths. A wooden stage was set up specifically for the dancers. Professional dancers were hired to dance alongside the afflicted. Whenever people began to slow their pace or seemed ready to collapse from exhaustion, the musicians played more upbeat music, using fifes or drums. The logic behind this was, according to Waller, that people suspected the disease was caused by "putrefying blood cooking normally moist and cool brains,"[16] and it could be cured only if the dancers remained in motion.

Some people joined in without actually being ill. The sixteenth-century chronicler Specklin claimed that there were "many frauds trying to benefit from the situation"[17] since the towns' citizens were donating food and wine to the dance halls. Free food was a big draw if you had survived the scarcity of "the bad year." The entertainment was over quickly, though. Specklin claimed, of the dance halls and music, that, despite the townspeople's great efforts and good intentions, "all of this helped not at all."[18] The weaker dancers collapsed from strokes or heart attacks and had to be carried off the dance floor by family members.

Later in the summer of 1518 a notice in Strasbourg read:

There's been a strange epidemic lately
Going amongst the folk
So that many in their madness
Began dancing
Which they kept up day and night
Without interruption
Until they fell unconscious
Many have died of it[19]

The chronicle suggests that fifteen people were dying per day.

Realizing that their plan to cure compulsive dancing with more dancing was ineffective, the town authorities decided that the plague had been sent by God as punishment for *all* their sinful ways. This is notable because they took responsibility as a community, rather than just blaming the afflicted individuals. Gambling and prostitution were outlawed, and anyone who participated in those activities was exiled from the town, though only "for a time." Instead of providing public dance floors and excellent music, authorities decided that those stricken with the strange plague should stay inside. An official at the time wrote: "As the dancing disease did not want to end, the city council decided, that families should stay in their houses when a member was infected—to make sure that nobody else was infected. If one of their servants was affected, families had to keep them on their expenses somewhere or send them to St. Vitus. It was punished heavily."[20] They actually decreed that you had to take care of people, even lowly servants.

Dancing was also outlawed. The only exception was for "honorable people" who wanted to dance at weddings or "first mass." However, even those people were firmly instructed "on conscience" not to use tambourines or drums.

A note from the time by Sebastian Brant read: "Sadly at this time a horrible episode arose with sick . . . dancing persons, which has not yet stopped, Our lord councilors of the XXI turned to the honor of God and forbade, on pain of a fine of 30 shillings, that anyone, no matter who, should hold a dance until St. Michael's Day [September 29] in this city or its suburbs or in its whole jurisdiction. For by so doing they take away the recovery of such persons."[21]

For by so doing they take away the recovery of such persons. What a town!

It is lovely to see that all the edicts related to helping the suffering people. The community did not want their fellow neighbors to die and were experimenting on many fronts to help the afflicted. Today we *still* have outbreaks where we become so fearful for ourselves that we forget all about our neighbors. The people of Strasbourg were ahead of their time in their regard for one another.

What actually seemed to cure the sufferers? The fixation on sending people to the shrine of St. Vitus? Yes, it did! I bet you didn't see that coming! At least it did according to Specklin's description. After outlawing all the prostitutes and sinners "for a time," town authorities "sent many on wagons to St. Vitus [shrine] in Hellensteg, beyond Severne, and others got their own. They fell down dancing before his image. So then a Priest said mass over them, and they were given a little cross and red shoes, on which the sign of the cross had been made in holy oil on both the tops and the soles."[22] The color red might have been selected because in prior plague outbreaks victims had been unable to see or unable to tolerate the sight of the color red. Or it might have been selected because it seemed that their feet were on fire.

If you are interested in artistic responses: yes, the dancing plague is the inspiration for the story-ballet-movie *The Red Shoes* (1948), about a girl who puts on a pair of red shoes and cannot stop dancing.

Not in this case, though!

After their pilgrimage to the shrine, many of the afflicted simply stopped dancing. They returned home and went back to their daily lives, probably somewhat worse for the wear, and forever afraid of drums and tambourines. Records state that the time at St. Vitus's shrine "helped many, and they gave a large contribution."[23]

It seems remarkable that dancing around a saint's shrine and wearing red shoes served as an effective cure because, as modern people, we know that diseases are not treated by magic. This isn't a matter of not having religious faith. It's a matter of not believing in vengeful saints cursing people and then curing them in exchange for donations to their shrines. Yet in the sixteenth century people really *did* believe in religious miracles, exorcisms, and transformations, in a way that we simply don't today. Believing they were being cured by a great power might have been enough to actually cure them. The dancing plague of 1347 was supposedly halted by a priest holding open the mouth of each suffering person and shouting into their mouths, "Praise the true God, Praise the holy Ghost, get thee hence, thou damned and foredoomed spirit."[24] (When your boss suggests you try new ideas and think outside the box, you could consider yelling into your coworkers' mouths the next time you're stuck on a work problem.) We could think of this unswerving faith in God and saints as having a kind of placebo effect, which we still experience today.

Strasbourg officials made sure the plague stricken were taken to the highest authority figure available. Okay, the treatment worked because the problem was likely largely the result of a psychological disorder. But as much as their faith in the power of St. Vitus might have cured the dancers, it seems equally valid to say that the sufferers were—wait for it—*cured by the power of friendship*. Seriously. The people of Strasbourg were

exceedingly, abnormally kind to those afflicted. They didn't burn them at stakes. They didn't permanently cast them out of the community. Thought and concern went into considering ways to make them healthy again. People *cared* about them, so much so they used the community's limited resources on (totally misguided) ideas like hiring professional dancers to hang out and caper alongside the sufferers. They then attempted to limit their own dancing because they were afraid of impeding other town members' recovery. When you compare this behavior to people abandoning their loved ones in the middle of the night during the bubonic plague, the difference in the level of care is staggering. And this kindness

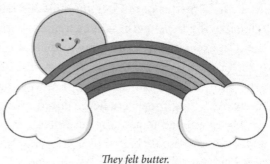

They felt butter.

may have been an overwhelming novelty for the sufferers. People were being nice to them, perhaps for the first time in what would have been their likely miserable lives. Waller writes that they might have been cured or at least unlikely to begin dancing again as

> many of them had experienced years of neglect, misery, want, and exploitation, but in the previous days or weeks they had been subject to the earnest attentions of civic and religious leaders who would normally have treated them with unmitigated contempt. To many of the alienated and the marginalized, the response of the authorities must have felt deeply gratifying. Reflecting on the assiduity with which Church

and government had sought to cure their ills, many were emotionally fortified against a relapse.[25]

Can we recover from a disease just by knowing that the people in charge *want* us to get better? Surely, government authorities *should* always want everyone to be healthy. Even if you assume government officials are all abject sociopaths, having people dying en masse in your town is bad PR. But it is rare, even today, that people suffering from diseases aren't demonized. The U.S. government sponsors antismoking ads, which often imply that smokers deserve to get lung cancer because they didn't quit smoking rather than putting those funds toward researching a cure for lung cancer, the actual enemy. Response to the AIDS crisis was delayed at least in part because those suffering were viewed by some as sinners. Clearly, those diseases take more than human kindness to cure, but there is never a situation where care and attentiveness by the community is a bad thing.

Hysterical outbreaks did not disappear after the sixteenth century. They still occur today. While the science behind them isn't fully understood, they are often thought to be related to terrible or repressive circumstances—the mind's confused and disordered attempt to make the conditions bearable. Mass hysteria is mainly associated with major trauma. For instance, Cambodians who survived the killing fields of the Khmer Rouge in the 1970s sometimes developed hysterical blindness. "Seventy percent of the women had their immediate family killed before their eyes," Professor Patricia Rozee-Koker of Cal State, Long Beach, told the *Los Angeles Times* when she was studying their vision complaints. "So their minds simply closed down, and they refused to see anymore—refused to see any more death, any more torture, any more rape, any more starvation."[26] Hysterical blindness had been a trope in war movies long before the

1970s. Usually a soldier would see something awful, go blind without any physical cause, and be nursed back to health by the love of a good woman. And though we might sneer at those movies and shout at the screen, "Medicine doesn't work that way!" I guess . . . sometimes someone being kind does make a difference to physical health.

In 1962 there was a laughing outbreak at a girls' school in Tanzania. It began with one girl laughing, then spread to the rest of the classroom, and then the entire school. It spread to at least 217 people. The girls alternated between laughing and crying, and became violent when the teachers demanded they stop. The affected girls would laugh and cry for about sixteen days, then stop, then start again. To this, you might say, "Well, that's an anomaly. Why would being a teenager in a girls' school be so psychologically unbearable?" Congratulations on becoming an adult who has utterly forgotten what it was like to be in high school.

Christian F. Hempelmann of Texas A&M, who studied the laughing epidemic, claimed that outbreaks of mass hysteria often begin when "there is an underlying shared stress factor in the population. It usually occurs in a group of people who don't have a lot of power."[27] Some people say that the outbreak in Tanzania might have occurred because the country had just become independent, and everyone in the community was under a tremendous amount of stress. But there are still instances of the laughing hysteria in Tanzania today. One woman recounted to the program RadioLab that it happened to three girls in her high school class the morning of a math exam.[28] One of the girls recovered only when her boyfriend came to stay with her in the hospital. If your immediate reaction is that she was faking illness to make a man pay attention, remember that people thought the same of Frau Troffea until she danced her feet off.

And, lest you're inclined to think, *Well, that couldn't happen here,* Waller notes: "Nor is the secular West invulnerable to hysterical fears. In fact, some are virtually endemic. American and to some extent European cultures remain awash with paranoid delusions of alien abduction and flying saucers."[29]

In 2012 a group of teenage girls from Le Roy, New York, began to simultaneously develop tics that caused them to twitch uncontrollably. Once the event was labeled as a bout of mass hysteria, it prompted one of their guardians to remark to the *New York Times Magazine,* "What are we—living in the 1600s?"[30] Though the doctors seemed to think the girls' symptoms were related to stresses in their lives, some did get better when put on antibiotics—which we have as much faith in as sixteenth-century Germans might have had in a shrine. (With good reason. The most terrifying medical problem we're likely to face in the near future is diseases becoming resistant to antibiotics.) Their doctor admitted to the *Times,* "It's hard to distinguish between the drug and the placebo effect."[31]

Today it often seems we consider physical wellness to be entirely separate from our emotional state. We like to think that Dr. House on television can be a great doctor despite the fact that he shouts at his patients things like, "You're barren, like a salt field!" or "So your kids committed suicide—get over it!" But treating patients unkindly does not mean that a doctor is smarter than everyone else; it just means that the doctor is emotionally deficient. It's perfectly possible to be smarter than everyone else and still be polite and even deferential—women have been doing it for centuries. Often people need the most tenderness when they are ill. Sometimes people actually need kindness to get well.

Human kindness counts.

There are, of course, going to be those who scoff at this notion, especially in the context of a book about diseases. Their scoffing changes nothing.

One explanation for mass hysteria, according to the *New York Times Magazine,* is that it is caused by "the maladaptive version of the kind of empathy that finds expression in actual physical sensation: the contagious yawn or sympathetic nausea or the sibling who grabs his own finger when he sees his brother's bleed."[32]

Of course diseases occur independent of mental states, but it is also true that given enough stress, people's internal miseries can manifest themselves physically. In a culture where being tough or cool means holding back most of your emotions almost all of the time, we are very used to suppressing loneliness or stress or sadness, and just deciding not to think about these feelings rather than admitting them. That's not an approach that works out really well. Extreme stress can manifest in real, physical, horrifying ways. It's great to deal with internal turmoil before you dance your feet off. And if you feel you might, talk to someone, who may or may not be a doctor.

We are good at treating people with medicine. It's one of the most amazing, magical accomplishments of the modern world. But that doesn't mean that people don't sometimes require more than medicine. We can all tend to our medicinal gardens, but we can also tend to one another. That's why every person in this chapter who came up with some crazy recovery plan or religious cure, or who just didn't believe the people in question were faking, qualifies as a hero in my book.

Smallpox

I was nauseous and tingly all over. I was either in love or I had smallpox.

—WOODY ALLEN

The impact of the Black Death on European nations from the fourteenth to the seventeenth century is remembered as one of the more horrifying chapters in history. However, European civilization endured. Some of the greatest artistic accomplishments in the Western world coexisted with the plague. Shakespeare's brother and sisters and his son died of the bubonic plague. Theaters were closed due to the plague during his lifetime. Hans Holbein and Titian painted great works before their deaths from the plague. Would they have preferred to live in a time without the Black Death? Yes. (This is not speculative. I called them all and asked.) But life went on in the face of death. Even the Roman Empire was able to endure for a few hundred years after the Antonine plague. Commodus was able to dither around killing ostriches.

So you might say, "Plague is not such a big deal, then, really." To which a more compassionate person might reply, "You know, we'll never read the plays Shakespeare's son might have produced." To be fair, they probably wouldn't have been that good. When children of famous people try to follow in their parents' footsteps, the output is decidedly mixed. However, I imagine a good bit of genius and human accomplishment were lost to the bubonic plague, even if European society did not completely collapse.

But if your definition of a big deal is the total destruction of a civilization, here is a plague for you. After being exposed to smallpox, the Aztec and Incan societies were devastated almost instantly. One year they were among the greatest civilizations in the world. The next year they basically *didn't exist.*

A front-runner in "historical outcomes you would not expect" was Francisco Pizarro's defeat of the Inca monarch Atahualpa—who was regarded as a god—in 1532. Atahualpa had an army of eighty thousand soldiers; Pizarro had a force of 168 men, of whom only 62 had horses.[1] Not only did the Spanish army kill seven thousand Incan soldiers the first night, Pizarro supposedly captured Atahualpa within *minutes.* After he did so, he promised Atahualpa, "We treat our prisoners and conquered enemies with mercy and only make war on those who make war on us. And, being able to destroy them, we refrain from doing so, but rather pardon them."[2] Anyone who has read about the Spaniards' treatment of native populaces during this period will recognize this statement as being the opposite of true. I can't even call it a lie, because there are plenty of big-fish stories and friendly white lies that are *not the precise opposite of everything your society has ever done.* Pizarro then demanded an entire room—twenty-two feet long by seventeen feet wide—full of gold in exchange for Atahualpa's life. The Incas peacefully provided the gold in the hope that the Spaniards would take it and leave. Pizarro then killed Atahualpa. Before the monarch died he promised to convert to Christianity if only the Spaniards would not burn him at the stake, as Incas believed that if a body was burned it could not ascend to the afterlife. They strangled him. Then, after he was dead, they set fire to his corpse.

All that in spite of the fact that, of the Incas, conquistador Pedro Cieza de León wrote: "Had [Pizarro] wished to convert [the Incas] with kind words, this people were so gentle and peaceful that all he needed was those few people with him and he could have done it."[3]

Between the conquistadores and the Spanish Inquisition, the Spaniards have a strong history of "doing unimaginably terrible stuff" through the sixteenth century. Christopher Buckley, in *But Enough About You,* describes the Spaniards' general attitude: "What an excellent time we shall have kidnapping, torturing and burning the Incas alive, to say nothing of raping their women, looting the country and destroying the last of a seven-thousand-year-old line of civilizations—all in the name of the One True Faith!"[4]

My favorite story about the Spaniards' horrific relationship to Amerindians comes from John Campbell's *An Account of the Spanish Settlements in America.* In this eighteenth-century report Campbell relays how the Spaniards reached Cuba in the sixteenth century and committed "the most horrid barbarities ever to taint the page of history." Before burning one native at the stake, a Spanish friar told him "that if he would embrace their religion he would go to heaven, but if not he would burn in hell forever." The Cuban asked if there were any Spaniards in heaven. The friar responded that there were. The Cuban replied, "If it be so, I would rather be with the devils in hell."[5]

Sick burn, Cuban guy. Nicely done—high five through time and space.

Now that everyone, including us and Christopher Buckley, is very clear that the Spaniards behaved deplorably in regard to America's native populace, we can ask how they won such a mismatched battle with the Incas and went on to take over the entire region.

The Spaniards had their own opinions on their success. At the time they seemed to think their unlikely victory was due to the fact that they were *excellent* Christians. They were zealous and devout. The message that Pizarro's brothers sent back to King Charles of Spain explained their victory over the Incas: "[It was] not accomplished by our own forces, for there were so few of us. It was by the Grace of God, which is great."[6]

I strongly suspect that sixteenth-century Spaniards merely skimmed the numerous "don't be awful people" portions of the Bible.

A more secular explanation for their victory is that the Spaniards had horses and guns and the Incas did not. The equipment certainly helped, but it's a stretch to believe that this factor alone would have been adequate against such a large Incan force. For some perspective: 168 people are about the number that a typical Chili's restaurant can accommodate. Hand all those diners guns—in addition to southwestern eggrolls and fire-grilled corn guacamole because it's going to be that kind of

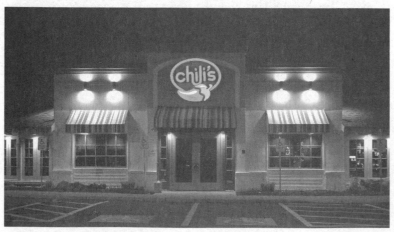

Hold this fortress at any cost.

night—and tell them they're going to be fighting a mob of eighty thousand people just outside. You might persuade them to join in this bold adventure if they are all extremely religious and you tell them God *wants* them to do this, but I think they'd still be scared. And remember you are giving them the kind of guns the Spaniards were using at the time, which took forever to load. I just don't think the diners at Chili's are going to be enthusiastic. I expect they might wish, in retrospect, that they had stayed home and ordered in.

Even the fervently religious Spaniards at the time understood that the odds were against them. They were scared. One of Pizarro's companions wrote: "The Indians' camp looked like a very beautiful city. They had so many tents that we were all filled with great apprehension. Until then, we had never seen anything like this in the Indies. It filled all our Spaniards with fear and confusion."[7] Even if they did credit the victory to God, many Spaniards seemed to think it was a weird fluke that they won such a mismatched battle. Especially because Pizarro had waged similar expeditions against the Incas in 1524 and 1526 and found that his army was too small and weak for effective combat against them.

The better explanation for their victory than God intervening on behalf of a bloodthirsty conquering army or the Spaniards' semi-okay guns and horses was the extent to which the Incas had been devastated by the arrival of smallpox. As the journalist Charles Mann writes: "So complete was the chaos [surrounding the smallpox outbreak] that Francisco Pizarro was able to seize an empire the size of Spain and Italy combined with a force of 168 men."[8]

Victory didn't hinge on guns and horses. It hinged on one man. A lone diseased Spaniard is believed to have introduced smallpox to the Incan society around 1525.

Today we know that smallpox is caused by the Variola virus. Once someone is infected they develop a fever—up to 104 degrees—which is sometimes accompanied by vomiting. Then they break out in a rash, which turns into bumpy pustules filled with clear liquid or pus. These later crust over and fall off, leaving pox marks on the skin.

Now, that description makes the disease sound unsightly but not deadly. Chicken pox (which is caused by a different virus) bears some resemblance and very rarely kills anyone. Meanwhile, smallpox is generally fatal in about 30 percent of the people it infects—though it would kill far more Amerindians. The best we understand it, the very condensed explanation for this death rate, which a wonderful doctor friend of mine provided, is that "smallpox makes your immune system go nuts. You die because your immune system kills you." The technical term is an uncontrolled immune response. Your immune system identifies an intruding virus or bacteria and, in its attempt to rid the body of the danger, freaks out. Chemicals are released in the bloodstream to fight the infection and trigger inflammation throughout the body. Organs are compromised and may shut down. If your immune system attacks your heart and your heart stops pumping blood effectively, your cells don't get oxygen. You die. If it attacks your kidneys, your blood can't be purified. You die.

The chicken pox virus doesn't generally provoke such a violent response in the body. It mostly just hangs out relatively harmlessly in your cells, sometimes causing new symptoms years later. If you love thinking in metaphorical terms, you could consider your body as a house and the chicken pox virus as an unpleasant former bandmate who wants to crash in your guest room indefinitely. The smallpox virus, however, is Godzilla. If Godzilla was suddenly inside your house, authorities (your immune system) would probably freak out and might firebomb the whole thing in an attempt to get rid of him. Deadbeat chicken pox is uncomfortable, but authorities aren't going to do much about it. He (chicken pox) is just going to live there, eating your food, having sex on your couch, and drinking your beer *forever.* You'll probably forget he's there after a while.

In some cases smallpox also causes a condition called disseminated intravascular coagulation (DIC). There are lots of little proteins in your body called *clotting factors* that cause your blood to coagulate, which stops you from bleeding to death every time you cut yourself shaving. If DIC occurs, those clotting factors come and start forming little tiny blobs in your bloodstream. Then more clotting factors join, and the blobs become bigger. The end result is that your blood stops clotting normally. You begin bleeding from abnormal places. And if the blobby clots get too big, blood cannot flow properly and your cells do not receive oxygen. Again, you die.

Prior to the outbreak of smallpox, the Inca civilization was thriving, in large part due to the ruler Huayna Capac. When he assumed control in 1493, the empire was already enormous. It stretched from Argentina all the way up to Colombia—encompassing about half of South America. Huayna Capac visited each province to meet with the governors. He oversaw repairs of infrastructure—like irrigation systems—and encouraged the planting of new crops like peanuts and cotton. During this time he commanded over fifty-five thousand troops and waged several victorious campaigns. Drawings from the period depict him being carried into battle on a litter covered in jewels. The great palace Quispiguanca was built as his hunting lodge, a kind of sixteenth-century South American Versailles, and there he partied and gambled with his favorite courtiers and generals. Meanwhile his wife amused herself tending to a flock of doves.[9] (This detail about the doves isn't really important. It just strikes me as a nice, civilized image. A dove is the most refined pet I can imagine.)

It was a good time to be Incan!

But that was before smallpox began to afflict the empire. Huayna Capac died of the disease in 1527. So did all of his favorite generals and most of his family. Supposedly on his deathbed Huayna Capac named his infant son as his heir, but by the time he did so, that baby had died as well. Then Huayna Capac said, "My father the sun is calling me. I shall go to rest by his side," which are very poetic last words. Unfortunately, better last words would have been a definitive statement on the order of succession. People couldn't decide whether Huayna Capac would have rather seen the country ruled by his legitimate son, Huáscar, or his favorite illegitimate son, Atahualpa.

Obviously, any confusion about who is going to rule is not desirable. It leads to civil wars. But dynastic squabbles were common among the Incas, and the people would have been happy with whoever emerged victorious in battle as their ruler. Huáscar and Atahualpa assembled armies, and a bitter civil war began to determine who would succeed Huayna Capac. Unfortunately, this war killed off many of their warriors while more were falling victim to smallpox. The Incas were experiencing great numbers of fatalities on two fronts. It is believed that if Huayna Capac had lived, even with the plague afflicting the Incas, the Spaniards would never have triumphed. Pizarro himself admitted: "If Huayna Capac had been alive when we invaded Peru, we could not have won for he was greatly loved by his people . . . We could neither have invaded nor triumphed—not even if over a thousand Spanish troops had come at once."[10] Once again: Having a brilliant, beloved leader at the helm of a country when the land is in turmoil is one of the best situations people can hope for. That becomes apparent when that leader is dead.

By the time Pizarro met and defeated Atahualpa's troops in 1532, they had been grievously weakened by war and disease. It's still remarkable that Pizarro's tiny band of men won, but maybe your fellow Chili's warriors would be more optimistic about their chances for survival if you told them that they would be facing a mob that was malnourished, exhausted, and very ill from a disease that had killed their leader and caused a civil war, but was one you had most likely already become immune to after suffering through it in childhood.

Smallpox also beset the other great American empire of the time, the Aztecs, who were settled in what is now Mexico. When a Spanish company, led by Hernán Cortés, arrived in 1519, they brought smallpox with them.

With the benefit of hindsight, the Aztecs should have immediately sprung into battle against the Spaniards. Instead, when Cortés's forces arrived in the Aztec capital of Tenochtitlan, they were welcomed in the way that American forces today expect to be greeted anytime they go anywhere. The Aztec leader Montezuma II showered Cortés with gifts, including beautiful necklaces of precious jewels, gold, and feathers.

This warm welcome wasn't extended because the Aztecs were as "gentle and peaceful" a people as the Incas. The Aztecs were—there is no way to get around this—generally described as bloodthirsty maniacs who practiced cannibalism and daily human sacrifice.

Let us digress for a small gory moment to talk about human sacrifice. Aztecs weren't alone in this practice. The Incas sacrificed humans as well—they just went about it in a sort of civilized way. Children, often chosen for their beauty, who were raised to be eventual preteen and teenage sacrifices for the community, were given high social status. They dined on special foods (like maize) that members of the lower classes couldn't enjoy. Before they went to their deaths, they were given a great feast in their honor and a personal meeting with the emperor. One sacrifice supposedly claimed, "You can finish with me now because I could not be more honored than by the feasts which they celebrated for me in Cuzco."[11] Afterward, they would be given drugs and alcohol and led up a mountain, where they would be knocked on the back of the head and left to die of exposure. Their families would be considered honored people for their sacrifice.

Two points: (1) I am not defending Incan human sacrifice just because the feast sounds like fun and (2) a historical YA novel from the perspective of such a doomed teenager would be a very good premise. I will likely not sue you if you steal this idea. I will, however, expect to be invited to the book party, which must be as good as that feast in Cusco.

Aztecs, on the other hand, would tie people to rocks each day and rip out their still-beating hearts, believing that this was necessary to keep the sun burning. They'd then kick the bodies down the temple stairs and, depending upon the source of information, allegedly eat the corpses. It was "considered a good omen if [the victims] cried a lot at the time of sacrifice."[12] To my fellow late risers: if every Aztec could have slept in until noon even one day, they would have realized the sun rose without requiring still-beating hearts, and countless lives would have been saved. Remember this the next time anyone criticizes your sleeping habits.

So Cortés wasn't welcomed in a surprisingly friendly fashion because the Aztecs were nice guys. It is instead likely—and most fortuitous—that he was warmly received because the timing of his arrival fell perfectly in line with prophecies regarding the return of the Aztec god Quetzalcoatl, a nice-ish deity who only required sacrifices of hummingbirds and butterflies. When the group of strange men on horseback, impressively firing guns, arrived at the same time as the expected coming of the god, some of the Aztecs were, at least temporarily, understandably confused.

Shortly after their arrival, Cortés's men imprisoned Montezuma II. However, when the Spaniards tried to seize Tenochtitlan they were met with formidable resistance by the city's forces, who supposedly proceeded to stone their leader to death because of his bad judgment with the feathers and gold and other gifts. From six hundred to one thousand conquistadores died in the ensuing battle—so many that June 30, 1520, came to be known as La Noche Triste (the Night of Tears or the Night of Sorrows). The Spaniards fled, and the Aztecs rejoiced. Their new leader, Cuauhtémoc, decided never to welcome strangers who are unproven gods into the city again, and life in Tenochtitlan returned to normal for about ten minutes.

The Spaniards weren't with the Aztecs long enough to capture the city, but they were—you guessed it—able to leave smallpox behind. One of Cortés's infected soldiers died during the battle, and his body was looted. The disease spread through the empire and devastated it. By September 1520 the inhabitants of Tenochtitlan had developed racking coughs and painful burning sores.[13] One Aztec account described what was called "the great rash": "Sores erupted on our faces, our breasts, our bellies, we were covered with agonizing sores from head to foot . . . the sick were so utterly helpless they could only lie on their beds like corpses, unable to move their limbs or even their heads. They could not lie facedown or roll from one side to the other. If they did move their bodies, they screamed in pain."[14] Aztec cities like Texcoco, which was estimated to have fifteen thousand citizens before the plague, would be left with only six hundred people, or 4 percent of its former population, by 1580.[15] Smaller towns and villages would simply be obliterated. Today, it's estimated that smallpox killed around 90 percent of the native people of the Americas.[16]

Even in Europe, where the disease was known, smallpox was terrifying because it was so contagious. Ole Didrik Lærum, a modern-day professor of medicine at the University of Bergen, claimed that "sometimes being in a room next door to someone who was infected was all it took."[17] Smallpox was even more terrifying and deadly to people who had never experienced it. One Spanish priest graphically described that the Aztecs "died in heaps, like bedbugs. In many places it happened that everyone in a house died and, as it was impossible to bury the great number of dead, they pulled down the houses over them so that their homes become their tomb."[18]

When Cortés returned in 1521, he was able to take the Aztec capital with ease. In addition to disease, "many died only of hunger . . . for they had no one left to look after them . . . No one cared about anyone else."[19] Sahagún, the friar and author of *Historia General*, who would claim to have buried ten thousand people before he died of smallpox himself in 1590, said that people lived in terror of any contact with their neighbors, much as Europeans had during the bubonic plague (which only killed 30 percent of the people in Europe). Sahagún worried that "the [Aztec's] land would revert to wild beasts and wilderness"[20] as there were too few Spaniards to settle it, and the Aztecs would soon be extinct. The few remaining Aztecs began a new calendar, which counted time anew from the year they first experienced "the Great Leprosy." This makes sense. The disease was so devastating, and the obliteration so complete, that their entire world could only be grouped as what came before and what came after.

Like the Aztecs, the Incas felt their world similarly altered. They recounted the arrival of smallpox in a mythic manner, as if it were a vengeful genie released from a bottle. In the 1613 *Antiquities of Peru*, J. de Santa Cruz Pachacuti-Yamqui Salcamayhua writes of the Incan telling of the beginning of the plague:

> There came a messenger with a black cloak, and he gave the Inca a kiss with great reverence, and he gave him a "pputi," a small box with a key. And the Inca told the same Indian to open it, but he asked to be excused saying that the Creator had commanded that only the Inca should open it.
>
> Understanding the reason why, the Inca opened the box, and there came fluttering out things like butterflies or scraps

of paper, and they scattered until they vanished. And this was the smallpox plague.[21]

Anyone familiar with Greek mythology will see the similarity between this tale and the story of Pandora's box. In that story, the first woman on earth opens a box that releases all the evils in the world, which fly out like insects. However, she manages to squeeze it shut just in time to keep hope from flying away as well.

There is no hope in the Incan story. There is only death. Pachacuti-Yamqui Salcamayhua's story ends: "Within two days the general Mihicnaca Mayta died, with many other distinguished captains, all their faces all covered with burning scabs. And when the Inca saw this, he ordered a stone house to be prepared for him in which to isolate himself. And there he died."[22] This ending seems considerably less mythological than the first part of the story.

The Spaniards shrugged off the horrors and devastation of the plague, saying, as Pedro Cieza de León did, "But the matters of the Indies are the judgments of God, and come from His profound wisdom, and He knows why He permitted what happened."[23]

That is . . . not a satisfying answer. Why were the effects of smallpox *so* devastating to these empires? In large part, the high death toll occurred because the Amerindians, prior to the arrival of European visitors, had absolutely no exposure to the kind of diseases that sixteenth-century Europeans considered a normal part of life. Therefore, they had no resulting immunities. That's not to say that smallpox wasn't a scourge in Europe as well; it killed around four hundred thousand people—many of them children—each year in Europe well into the eighteenth century.[24] But those surviving the disease developed immunity, and a small degree of immunity could be passed down through parents.

Smallpox is thought to have originated with farm animals—especially cattle, but also horses and sheep—and then crossed species to infect humans. Europeans had a great deal of contact with those animals, whereas the Inca and Aztec people had none. As Jared Diamond, the author of *Guns, Germs and Steel*, explains: "The Incas had llamas, but llamas aren't like European cows and sheep. They're not milked, they're not kept in large herds, and they don't live in barns and huts alongside humans. There was no significant exchange of germs between llamas and people."[25] The devastation of smallpox in the Americas was not due to a vengeful God or a mysterious man bearing an evil box, but rather to the fact that Amerindians did not spend as much quality time with their domesticated llamas as Europeans did with their cows.

Now, maybe you are reading these tales of destruction and thinking, *Oh, God, I myself do not have a cattle farm*, or *I am a proud llama farmer* (there's got to be one *somewhere*), and are therefore convinced that you would surely die if you contracted smallpox because of your sad immune system—and what if terrorists purposefully incubate smallpox and come in a suicidal pact and spread it to us, and we *all die* and our civilization *perishes* and everything is *very bad*? I am with you, citizen! Considering what happened to the Romans and the Amerindians, an outbreak of smallpox is an extremely frightening prospect. Fortunately, the World Health Organization officially declared the disease eradicated worldwide in 1979. Accordingly, we are no longer even vaccinated to prevent it. However, after September 11, 2001, the U.S. government became as concerned as you might be right now. It stockpiled enough vaccine to protect every person in the United States, and the vaccine is effective within three days of being exposed to the disease. Worst-case scenario: if some very evil people unleashed smallpox into the general population, there is a plan in place to prevent many casualties. So though smallpox is a very scary disease, it's not one we need to be especially fearful of today.

This desirable state of affairs is largely thanks to Edward Jenner. In the eighteenth century the English doctor and scientist realized that milkmaids who had suffered from cowpox—a disease which results in only a few small sores on the hands—never contracted smallpox. He began injecting people who were not milkmaids with a small amount of pus from cowpox blisters, in an attempt to ensure that they too would never suffer smallpox. Now, there were people before him who had attempted a similar (though less safe) procedure. A medical paper titled "The Myth of the Medical Breakthrough: Smallpox, Vaccination, and Jenner Reconsidered" asserts: "It is extremely rare that a single individual or experiment generates a quantum leap in understanding; his 'lone genius' paradigm is potentially injurious to the research process."[26] I don't think that's necessarily true. I love lone geniuses! I love heroes, and I will take them any way I can, because it's inspiring to imagine one person hauling all of humanity forward.

But in this case, Jenner metaphorically stood on the pox-touched shoulders of harem girls and Lady Mary Wortley Montagu.

As far back as ancient Roman times, it was understood that people who had survived smallpox once did not get the disease again. Having already read about the kind of "cures" attempted for the bubonic plague, you can guess that this basic knowledge of immunity didn't stop people in Europe from developing some alternative theories about how to treat the disease. In the seventeenth century Dr. Thomas Sydenham recommended "twelve bottles of small beer every twenty-four hours,"[27] which I suppose at least temporarily distracted the patients from their disfiguring pox and made them feel confident about their ability to heal and look more attractive than ever. As, doubtless, did the fact that Sydenham believed in prescribing opium for everything.

While Europeans were guzzling beer, a technique known as *variolation* became popular in the Ottoman Empire. Variolation generally entailed finding someone suffering from smallpox, drawing blood or fluid from one of their pustules, and injecting it into an uninfected person. Other methods of transfer might include rubbing infected bits of scab on open wounds or snorting smallpox crusts up your nose. The uninfected person would usually develop the disease but in a less severe form than if they had contracted it naturally. They would get *a little bit* sick rather than *a lot* sick, and hopefully recover with minimal damage. In the Turkish empire, as early as 1600, variolation was frequently performed on young girls who were being considered for the sultan's harem. The injection would be done on parts of the body where, even if there were some scarring, it would be less likely to mar their beauty.

Which was important in a harem girl, obviously. Smallpox was a killer, but it was also referred to as "beauty's enemy." Sahagún, in reference to the Aztec outbreak, wrote: "Many who came down lost their good looks, they were deeply pitted and remained permanently scarred. Some lost their sight and became blind."[28]

The women in Turkey who were variolated would experience less disfigurement, but there were still downsides. For one thing, they were perhaps going to have to live in a harem. Despite what nineteenth-century romantic paintings would have you believe, a harem was like a sorority house located in hell. On a more practical, disease-related note, harem dwellers could acquire all manner of blood diseases—like syphilis—from the variolation, or they could have *a severe reaction to the smallpox sample and die.* There was a 2 to 3 percent fatality rate from variolation. If a procedure had a one in fifty chance of killing you, the FDA would not look favorably upon it today. But the odds were certainly preferable to the much higher likelihood of death, blindness, or disfigurement from naturally contracted smallpox. For a group of women who would be living in close quarters and whose only means of gaining power was to be as beautiful and beloved by the sultan as possible, variolation may have been a very sound approach.

Lady Mary Wortley Montagu, whose husband was the British ambassador to the Ottoman Empire in 1716, would never have made it as a harem girl. Although Lady Mary had been famously beautiful, she had suffered from smallpox and her face was marked by it. If a woman's worth lay only with her beauty, as it did through much of history, contracting smallpox might seem to be a fate worse than death. Isobel Grundy, Lady Mary Montagu's biographer, notes, "Smallpox discourse was gendered, referring to men it spoke of the danger to life, referring to women, of the danger to beauty."[29] Women in Europe— and presumably all over the world—tried desperately and often in vain to recover their looks after surviving smallpox. A line in the 1696 play *Love's Last Shift* reads: "I take more pains to preserve a public reputation / than any lady took after the Smallpox to recover her complexion."[30]

When Lady Mary heard of the Turkish technique, she was fascinated and excited, reporting, "The French ambassador says pleasantly that they take the smallpox here by way of diversion as they do the waters in other countries."[31] She wrote of the process that she witnessed:

> The old woman comes with a nutshell full of the matter of the best sort of smallpox, and asks what vein you please to have opened. She immediately rips open that you offer to her, with a large needle (which gives you no more pain than a common scratch) and puts into the vein as much matter as can lie upon the head of her needle, and after that, binds up the little wound with a hollow bit of shell, and in this manner opens

four or five veins. The Grecians have commonly the superstition of opening one in the middle of the forehead, one in each arm, and one on the breast, to mark the sign of the Cross; but this has a very ill effect, all these wounds leaving little scars, and is not done by those that are not superstitious, who chuse to have them in the legs, or that part of the arm that is concealed. The children or young patients play together all the rest of the day, and are in perfect health to the eighth. Then the fever begins to seize them, and they keep their beds two days, very seldom three. They have very rarely above twenty or thirty [sores] in their faces, which never mark, and in eight days time they are as well as before their illness.[32]

Lady Mary didn't just latch on to a superstition. Instead she observed the effects of treatment on those around her. Although she did not benefit from the treatment, having already contracted smallpox, she had variolation performed (successfully) upon her two children. As word spread of the technique, it was tested in Newgate prison in 1721 on six inmates, who would each receive a pardon for submitting to the treatment. They all survived and were later found to be immune to smallpox.

By the end of the eighteenth century, variolation had become common throughout the world. King Frederick II of Prussia had all of his soldiers treated, as did George Washington at Valley Forge in 1778. People in France were more resistant to the procedure, causing the philosopher Voltaire to fume, "Had [variolation] been practiced in France it would have saved the lives of thousands."

Edward Jenner—*lone-ish genius and hero*—was himself variolated against smallpox as a child in the traditional way. But he was intrigued by a dairymaid he heard declare, "I shall never have smallpox for I have had cowpox. I shall never have an ugly pockmarked face." In 1796 Jenner found a milkmaid with cowpox and injected the matter from one of her sores into an eight-year-old boy, who developed a mild fever and a loss of appetite but recovered quite quickly. Ten days later, Jenner proceeded to inject the boy with actual smallpox. The boy survived! With no signs of smallpox. That experiment sounds terrifying, but it worked. Jenner called the technique *vaccination*, as *vacca* was the Latin word for "cow."

Cowpox vaccination was superior to smallpox variolation in that the vaccine from the less dangerous cowpox disease didn't kill *anybody* but still provided immunity. This was the first building block on the road to safe vaccines, which have since been developed for many life-threatening diseases. Polio. Measles. Meningitis. Diphtheria. We've triumphed over them all.

At the time, though, vaccination was controversial. Many were opposed.

In a 1911 issue of *American Magazine,* Sir William Osler, M.D., addressed the people who refused to vaccinate against smallpox:

> Here I would like to say a word or two upon one of the most terrible of all acute infections, the one of which we first learned the control through the work of Jenner. A great deal of literature has been distributed casting discredit upon the value of vaccination in the prevention of small-pox. I do not see how anyone who has gone through epidemics as I have, or who is familiar with the history of the subject, and who has any capacity left for clear judgement, can doubt its value. Some months ago I was twitted by the editor of the Journal of the Anti-Vaccination League for a "curious silence" on this subject. I would like to issue a Mount-Carmel-like challenge to any ten unvaccinated priests of Baal. I will go into the next severe epidemic with ten selected, vaccinated persons and ten selected unvaccinated persons—I should prefer to choose the latter—three members of Parliament, three anti-vaccination doctors (if they can be found), and four anti-vaccination

propagandists. And I will make this promise—neither to jeer nor jibe when they catch the disease, but to look after them as brothers, and for the four or five who are certain to die, I will try to arrange the funerals with all the pomp and ceremony of an anti-vaccination demonstration.[33]

That is the best, snarkiest denouncement of people who do not believe in vaccines I have ever read. I especially like the part where he asks to pick which politicians will die.

Today you may have heard from a vocal minority of people who do not believe in vaccination. Many of those people distrust vaccines because in 1998 a gastroenterologist named Andrew Wakefield published a paper in the *Lancet* claiming there was a link between children receiving the vaccine for measles, mumps, and rubella (MMR) and children developing autism.

Wakefield was a fraud. In 2010 he was stripped of his medical license. He was found to have conducted unethical experiments and accepted hundreds of thousands of dollars from lawyers attempting to sue the makers of MMR vaccines.[34] Wakefield was also attempting to create a new measles vaccine and would have profited handsomely if the MMR vaccine was discredited. He preyed upon people's fears and their concern for their children in order to obtain personal advantage. After an investigation by the intrepid *Sunday Times* journalist Brian Deer, it was found that the medical histories of all twelve children in Wakefield's study had been misrepresented.[35] In 2010 the editor of the *Lancet* issued the following retraction: "it was utterly clear, without any ambiguity at all, that the statements in the paper were utterly false."[36]

And yet many persist in believing Wakefield's conclusions.

So for people who do not wish to vaccinate their children, let me say that raising children seems very difficult. My job, as I see it, is to support my friends in their child-rearing decisions. They want to send their toddler off to a Swiss boarding school?

That's great! Four-year-olds who know how to play polo inspire not only admiration but terror, which in my mind means respect! They're going to let their daughter choose her own name and send her to a hippie academy where the students learn to draw instead of read? Also great! It sounds like Princess Jellybean Frostina Elsa will be very creative or, as she would write, "!!☺ ☺****☺!!"

The only time I think it is worth expressing anything other than support is if people are actively putting their children in danger. So if someone leaves their child vulnerable to deadly diseases like measles by not vaccinating, I will speak up. Parents refusing to vaccinate their children are doing something akin to allowing their kids to run about in traffic because they are irrationally afraid of sidewalks or they believe being struck by an oncoming car might be good in the long run. And it's not only their own children they are putting at risk. If you have children, they're also putting *your* children at risk. Vaccinating most of the population protects the very young and vulnerable people of all ages who cannot be safely vaccinated. And for those who think, for instance, measles, which we vaccinate against, is an antiquated disease they don't need to worry about, according to the World Health Organization it still kills nearly 115,000 people a year globally.[37] Vaccines don't result in hundreds of thousands of deaths. But they only work if everyone who can be is vaccinated. If one child gets measles because of a parent's foolishness, that child might risk infecting the children of better informed parents.

It seems that some antivaccination proponents are under the impression that the past was populated with beautiful, strapping men and women who had naturally robust immune systems made hardier because of their exposure to childhood diseases. Those people have watched too many movies. When you think of unvaccinated people, do not think of the hunks in the Starz TV series *Outlander* (2014). Those are today's actors *playing* old-timey people. (You can tell because they have all their teeth.) Think instead of the large numbers of people who were left blind from their exposure to smallpox. Or the people who were pockmarked for life. Or think instead of the Aztecs and the Incas, their civilizations decimated, their homes pulled down on their dead bodies. Think of what it might have been like when 30 to 90 percent of your friends and family died, because that was the world before vaccines. Ask the Aztecs and Incas whether or not they would have liked to have vaccines available to them. Oh, wait, you can't, they're dead.

Vaccination is one of the best things that has happened to civilization. Empires toppled like sandcastles in the wake of diseases we do not give a second thought to today. If taking a moment to elaborate on that point will make this book unpopular with a large group of antivaxxers, that's okay. This feels like a good hill to die on. It's surely a better one than the Incas got.

Syphilis

"WHORES.
Necessary in the nineteenth century for the contraction of
syphilis, without which no one could claim genius."

—*Flaubert's Parrot*, JULIAN BARNES

If you believe the many biographies of great men and women, none of them ever had syphilis.

Which would be a remarkable stroke of luck on their part. Since its discovery in Barcelona in 1493—supposedly brought back from the New World—the sexually transmitted disease just mowed down Europeans. Its effects were so devastating that some regard it as an equal trade for the measles and the smallpox Europeans exported to the Americas. The initial outbreak is estimated to have killed over one million Europeans, prompting the sixteenth-century artist Albrecht Dürer to write: "God save me from the French disease. I know of nothing of which I am so afraid . . . Nearly every man has it and it eats up so many that they die."[1]

To avoid syphilis, if you time travel to a year before 1928,

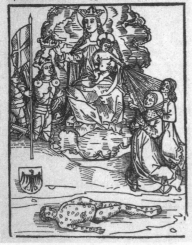

Tractatus de pestilentiali Scotra siue mala de Franzos. Origine Remediaq; eiusde cōtinens. cōpilatus a venerabili viro Magistro Joseph Grünpeck de Burckhausen. super Carmina quedā Sebastiani Brandt. vtriusq; iuris pfessoris.

This insane woodcutting shows baby Jesus merrily shooting syphilis rays at people like he's a comic book super-villain.

you should marry a very religious person who has never had sex. Also, you should never have sex, even with your spouse, for there's a chance he or she is untrustworthy and has had or is having extramarital sex, and will bring the disease back to your home, where your beloved will pass it to you. Just be a sexless but healthy person.

If you are thinking, *I am going to try, but I am not 100 percent certain I can live like that,* well, neither did anyone else in history. Even the Catholic Church fell into disgrace following the outbreak of syphilis in Europe as evidence of its symptoms began to mar the faces of the clergy.

Everybody (possibly a slight exaggeration) contracted syphilis. Really, just name a famous person between the years 1520 (when written records of the disease are first available) and 1928. They probably had syphilis. I will get you started . . . Beethoven is thought to have had it. So is Napoleon. Schubert almost certainly did. Flaubert definitely did. It's suspected that Hitler had it. Columbus is thought to have died from it. Even Mary Todd and Abraham Lincoln are believed to have had syphilis.

The fact that we may never know how widespread the disease actually was has a lot to do with the reluctance of sufferers to admit they had syphilis or to suggest others had it. Claims about how many people and specifically which individuals had syphilis are still controversial. For instance, many biographers dispute that Lincoln was syphilitic, despite his friend W. H. Herndon's report in 1891: "About the year 1835–36 Mr. Lincoln went to Beardstown and during a devilish passion had connection with a girl and caught the disease. Lincoln told me this and in a moment of folly I made a note of it in my mind."[2] I suppose there is a chance that longtime friends and business associates make up very specific lies about their friends' medical conditions because . . . well, who knows why people make stuff up? Maybe W. H. Herndon secretly *hated* Lincoln and his history of nice letters and kind words was just a long con. Still, I tend to believe actual acquaintances over people who live hundreds of years apart from the figures they profile. Some of those biographers are very invested in preserving the reputation of their heroes. When the explorer Meriwether Lewis's biographer, Stephen Ambrose, was asked by the *New York Times* if Lewis had syphilis, he primly replied, "Not even his biographer has a right to know that."[3] I think that, as a general rule, biographers should know what diseases their subjects had. Otherwise all biographies would conclude, "Then they died. Who knows why? I sure don't."

Part of that reluctance to label anyone as syphilitic likely has to do with the fact that the disease is called "the great imitator." Syphilis presents so many symptoms that it can be mistaken for numerous other diseases. More likely, though, that hesitance is because syphilis carried—and continues to bear—the stigma of being a sexually transmitted disease. STDs can often be the most difficult diseases to combat because no one wants to admit to having them. Why would you, when STDs are viewed by some as punishment for sin or lust? A recent health-care awareness campaign on Twitter encouraged those with STDs to #shoutyour status. Those brave enough to do so were met with responses like "If I had herpies [*sic*] I'd slit my arm open eat a bullet run in traffic . . . I hope you try at least one of these cures ☺ Sincerely 99% of the men in America."

That is the kind of response people get for saying that they have an irritating but not at all deadly sexually transmitted skin infection in 2016. (Also, if anyone sincerely, albeit bizarrely, believe that herpes is *a fate worse than death*, they should really be out trying to fund a cure and not yelling death threats at strangers online.)

No *wonder* people didn't want to talk about having syphilis. Which did not stop them from contracting it.

The means of transmission in the case of syphilis is simple. A syphilitic sore contains the spirochete bacterium *Treponema pallidum,* which can work its way into your body through mucous membranes, like those that line the anus, urethra (on a penis), vagina, or mouth—essentially every area of potential sexual contact. Syphilis first presents about three weeks after infection with a little sore (or sores) called a chancre (or chancres), which appears in the area where syphilis entered the body. That chancre is generally painless, and it will heal. Many people won't even notice it. However, five to twelve weeks after the sore has healed, patients often experience a fever or a rash (often on the palms of the hands and soles of the feet), which in some cases looks like chicken pox. The rash is usually painless, but it is extremely infectious, as any secretions contain the bacteria. This is a sign that syphilis is spreading through the body and will begin to affect the skin, lymph nodes, and brain.

If you have these symptoms, you have syphilis. Go to your doctor right away. Get a penicillin prescription. Make some phone calls to your past partners and go on with your life absolutely unimpeded.

One hundred years ago there was no penicillin, which was very unfortunate if you had syphilis.

After the initial stages, the disease enters a period of latency where the bacteria just hangs out in the spleen and lymph nodes. In some people, syphilis remains latent for decades. Those people are very lucky. However, for 15 to 30 percent of people who don't receive treatment, syphilis advances to the positively terrifying tertiary stage.[4] Symptoms can include joint problems and serious headaches. Sufferers' irises can become inflamed, leading to vision problems and sometimes blindness. Others might experience tremors and seizures. Some can become partially paralyzed. Many also develop a condition called *tabes dorsalis*, which causes intense, shooting pain throughout the body as the nerves along the spinal cords degenerate.

Neurosyphilis, when the disease invades the nervous system, can occur at any stage, though it's most often associated with tertiary syphilis. It involves an inflammatory response in the brain that leads to the destruction of bundles of nerve fibers. In some cases, the symptoms of neurosyphilis are mild, like headaches. However, many patients experience mental problems, like bouts of mania, changes in personality, and severe dementia. Sometimes, these mental problems lead to great creative outbursts. The philosopher Friedrich Nietzsche likely suffered from syphilis during his later period, when he wrote works such as *Ecce Homo* (1888). There's some controversy over whether he was syphilitic, because there is *always* controversy over whether someone was syphilitic. Except, weirdly, with regard to the composer Franz Schubert. His friends burned all of his letters and diaries after he died in an attempt to cover up his illness, and every biographer is still saying, "Yep, the one thing we're certain of is that guy *for sure* had syphilis."

Despite claims to the contrary, I am 99.9 percent sure Nietzsche had syphilis. As in the case of Schubert, Nietzsche's family engaged in a massive cover-up after his death. Nietzsche's extremely moralistic sister called the suggestion that he had syphilis a "disgusting suspicion."[5] Since then, neurologists have speculated that Nietzsche's madness might have been due to conditions ranging from CADASIL (an inherited stroke disorder) to a brain tumor. Finding alternate explanations for diseases seems like fun. But it's also absurd. Nietzsche was actually diagnosed with syphilis at the end of his life. That's rare to begin with because most people did everything possible to deny having the disease. But in the year 1889, eleven years before his death, Neitzsche was admitted to a clinic and officially diagnosed with syphilis (after admitting to himself that he'd been exposed to syphilis decades earlier). That seems to point very clearly toward his condition. He had a tiny scar on his penis from a healed syphilitic sore. And his mania, blindness, and illegible handwriting in his later letters, if they do not absolutely prove his illness, at least seem to do a very good imitation of syphilis's symptoms.

The psychiatrist Carl Gustav Jung later stated, "That exceedingly sensitive, nervous man had a syphilitic infection. That is a historical fact—I know the doctor who took care of him."[6] Jung made this claim when explaining his interpretation of one of Nietzsche's dreams wherein Nietzsche ate a toad in front of a lady. He reassuringly went on to say that if you have bad dreams, they aren't *necessarily* because you have been infected with a venereal disease. So that's good, and, also, let's conclude that Nietzsche did have syphilis because that is the correct conclusion.

The neurologist Sigmund Freud suspected the mania of syphilis could have benefited Nietzsche's work. Freud remarked: "It is the loosening process resulting from the paresis [syphilis-induced inflammation of the brain] that gave him the capacity for the quite extraordinary achievement of seeing through all layers and recognizing the instincts at the very base. In that way, he placed his paretic disposition at the service of science."[7]

Freud wasn't the only one who thought that having syphilis could allow for works of genius. The early twentieth-century poet Marc La Marche wrote in his poem "Syphilis":

> Are you not, Syphilis, the great go-between
> Working to put man in touch with his genius
> The source of powerful thoughts, the transmitter
> Of the seeds of art and science, the inspirer

Of delightful follies?
If we must put up crosses
To get them, we accept your laws
O Syphilis, salt of the earth!

This kind of glamorization is foolish. You know what no one ever says now? "Let's bring back syphilis because it makes people more creative!" If you want to be inspired, you don't contract a disease that's going to blind you and give you shooting pains all over your body. You just buy one of those books with bold, blocky print on the cover that explain how to have seven ideas every seven minutes.

In battle, when people are faced with a terrifying enemy, some think they can increase their chances of survival by defecting and befriending the enemy. You can't do that with a disease. You can't decide to be on its side in order to be spared or treated kindly by it. *And yet some people try.* Silver linings we attribute to diseases—whether those linings are that syphilitics have moments of manic genius, or tuberculosis sufferers become angelically beautiful, or people with Alzheimer's learn to live in the moment—are total bullshit. They do not lessen the horrors of the disease for anyone suffering from it. Instead they demean the very real suffering of victims and can make society less motivated to find a cure.

The way Nietzsche died was gruesome. He was institutionalized for mental illness brought on by syphilis. Although he was lucid for periods of time, during the last part of his life, the Oxford Roundtable Scholar Walter Stewart notes, "he drank urine, he ate feces, he saved feces, smeared feces on the walls and on himself."[8] The historian Deborah Hayden paints a similar picture: toward the end of his life, "he gesticulated and grimaced continually while speaking . . . he continued to be agitated and frequently incoherent. He smeared his feces and drank his urine. He screamed."[9] He was paraded in front of classes of medical students as a case study of what inflammation of the brain does to a person. What a horrific juxtaposition with the days when Nietzsche lectured in front of eager students as the youngest classics professor at the University of Basel. In his final days, Nietzsche was released from the clinic into his mother's care. His friend Franz Overbeck, who had earlier wondered if he should put Nietzsche out of his misery by euthanizing him, recalled their last meeting, when Nietzsche was huddled, "half crouching in a corner," desperate to be left alone.[10]

Nietzsche was one of the greatest philosophers of the twentieth century. And he was only age fifty-five when he died *in such a terrible way.*

Many syphilitics suffered similarly grim ends. The painter Theo van Gogh (the brother of Vincent) became violent in his dementia and attacked his wife and child. The author Guy de Maupassant lost his mind in a more gentle fashion and, in his last days, anxiously asked everyone if they knew where his thoughts had gone: "You haven't seen my thoughts anywhere, have you?" He believed they might be like butterflies that he could catch as they flitted through the air if he moved quickly enough. He ultimately had to be restrained and died murmuring, over and over, "the darkness, the darkness."[11]

There's no good way to die, but these seem like such stunningly dark ends for some of the brightest minds of their time.

The only upside might be that these victims still had lips to murmur with when they died. Another horrifying aspect of syphilis is that it could make your skin rot. In Upton Sinclair's novel about syphilis, *Damaged Goods*, a doctor describes the physical effects of the disease: "I have watched the spectacle of an unfortunate young woman, turned into a veritable monster by means of a syphilitic infection . . . Her face, or rather let me say what was left of her face, was nothing but a flat surface seamed with scars . . . Of the upper lip not a trace was left; the ridge of the upper gums appeared perfectly bare."[12] *And that doesn't even mention what the disease did to noses.*

Sufferers of syphilis developed a "saddle nose." The bridge of their nose would cave in—giving it the curved appearance of a saddle. This may not sound like that big a deal, but the rest of the flesh, say, around the nostrils, would also rot away, so they might be left with just the tip of their (decaying) nose exposed.

Just as those on #shoutyourstatus today are bombarded with messages telling them they are undeserving of respect, noseless people of the past were not treated with kindness. In the 1890 text *Surgical Experience Dealing Especially with the Reconstruction of Destroyed Parts of the Human Body Using New Methods,* the surgeon Johann Friedrich Dieffenbach wrote: "A blind man arouses pity, but a person without a nose creates repulsion and horror. And what's more, the world is still used to regarding this unfortunate disfigurement as a punishment . . . the unfortunate man who has lost his nose enjoys no pity at all, least of all from bigots, homeopaths, and hypocrites."[13]

Unsurprisingly, many sufferers wore a metal or wooden nosepiece to cover the rot so that people wouldn't draw back in horror. Those nosepieces were often connected to an early prototype of sunglasses, which were useful, as syphilis also causes its victims to become extremely sensitive to light.

For those looking for a more permanent solution, a technique called *paramedian forehead nasal flap reconstruction* was sometimes used. With this surgery, which had been practiced in India from 600 BC but only became popular in England in the early nineteenth century, a flap of skin was cut from the forehead and sutured onto the donor site, in this case, the nose. For syphilitics, the skin of the forehead was used because it matched the skin of the nose. Are you are thinking, *Did this look great after completion?!* No, of course not. The procedure often resulted in extremely weird eyebrow positioning, though that is better than having no nose. That said, recipients had to be careful afterward. Their new nose could fall off if they had an especially violent sneezing fit.[14]

Other surgeons attempted an "Italian" procedure invented by the surgeon Gaspare Tagliacozzi. It involved grafting skin from the arm rather than the forehead. The sixteenth-century doctor Leonardo Fioravanti described the process: "They snipped the skin on the arm at one end and sewed it to the nose. They bound it there so artfully that it could not be moved in any way until the skin had grown onto the nose. When the skin flap was joined to the nose, they cut the other end from the arm. They skinned the lip of the mouth and sewed the flap of skin from the arm onto it . . . It's a fine operation and an excellent experience."[15] "An excellent experience"! In *The Professor of Secrets: Mystery, Medicine, and Alchemy in Renaissance Italy,* the historian William Eamon writes, "one can only imagine what excruciating agony the operation must have caused."[16] The arm was held in a brace to keep it connected to the nose for a process that often took *forty days* to complete. Yet, in spite of this torturous approach, when Fioravanti visited the surgeon performing the operation, there were five patients waiting in line for the procedure.

Naturally, sufferers wanted to actually prevent and cure their disease and avoid creating some flimsy Mr. Potato Head–type nose out of skin from somewhere else on their body. Condoms were created in the sixteenth century specifically to fend off syphilis, but they were expensive and often reused several times, making them ineffective.

There were a few other treatments available before penicillin was officially recognized as an effective cure in 1947. In 1519 the German scholar Ulrich von Hutten wrote in *De Morbo Gallico* about the frequent use of the guaiacum plant to treat the symptoms of syphilis. He wasn't entirely wrong—the plant does have medicinal properties. Today it is used to treat sore throats. The expectorant guaifenesin, found in most cough syrups, is derived from it. Doctors from the past weren't necessarily idiots. Many of them were good at figuring out which plants and potions worked in some capacity; sadly, these findings usually fell short of actually curing people.

Imagine, today, how you would feel if your doctor could only give you cough syrup for every ailment. And if, when you protested, he said, "No, seriously, this is the best we've got. Good luck." Let's now take a minute to appreciate what it means to live in the modern era.

Despite liberal use of the guaiacum plant, and claims that it had cured him painlessly, von Hutten died from complications of tertiary syphilis in 1523.

His approach, however, did provide an alternative to mercury treatments, used liberally from the sixteenth century into the twentieth century. Mercury therapies were recommended by our old acquaintance/nemesis from the dancing plague chapter, Paracelsus. The treatments were so popular that people joked, "A night with Venus, a lifetime with mercury." In "Syphilis: The Great Pox," S. V. Beck describes a version of the treatment: "A patient undergoing the treatment was secluded in a hot, stuffy room, and rubbed vigorously with the mercury ointment several times a day. The massaging was done near a hot fire, which the sufferer was then left next to in order to sweat. This process went on for a week to a month or more, and would later be repeated if the disease persisted."[17]

But mercury is poisonous. Excessive exposure to mercury causes skin to peel; hair, teeth, and nails to fall out; and insanity. The term *mad hatters* comes from the fact that nineteenth-century hat makers were often exposed to and indeed went mad from mercury fumes. Mercury—whether rubbed on, ingested through a pill, or injected as became popular in the eighteenth and nineteenth centuries—cannot make you "healthy." In 1812 a "clinical test" was carried out, where British soldiers with syphilis were given mercury treatments, and Portuguese soldiers with syphilis were given none. The Portuguese soldiers had fewer health problems. Admittedly, that could be attributable to other factors. Maybe those Portuguese soldiers were just very hardy! However, an Oslo study conducted on two thousand syphilitics from 1891 to 1910 had similar results, finding that 60 percent of patients in the study who were not treated with mercury experienced fewer negative complications than those who had been.[18]

The reason von Hutten preferred guaiacum was that complications from mercury treatments could be so severe. As the medical historian Lawrence I. Conrad explains, "Von Hutten describes the distress and pain of the mercury treatment with its effusions of sweat and saliva, and the heat of the sweat-room in which patients suffocated, their throats so constricted that they could not vomit their own mucus."[19] So mercury treatments were painful, time-consuming, and ultimately detrimental to the sufferer's health.

One primitive method of treating syphilis that did technically work was raising a person's body temperature to an extreme degree. However, for the syphilis bacteria to die, the patient's temperature has to be raised to 107 degrees, which can result in major organ failure and seizures. If body temperature rises to 108 degrees, the person will die, along with the syphilis bacteria. So there's not a lot of room for error, and that "exactly 107 degrees" temperature is hard to hit without the aid of modern technology. Another approach was considered in 1917, when Julius Wagner-Jauregg attempted to inject syphilitics with malaria to cause a high fever and then cure them with quinine. He won the Nobel Prize for his work, but he also killed around 15 percent of his patients. And then there were arsenic-based treatments—such as the "magic bullet," Salvarsan. Arsenic treatments could work but often produced toxic side effects. Because arsenic is a poison.

Reading about all of these well-meaning but certainly dangerous attempts at a cure, I sometimes think the treatment for syphilis consisted of "trying things so terrifying that the disease is literally scared out of your body."

Perhaps the most terrible aspect of syphilis—even worse than chopping off part of your arm to give yourself a fake nose—was the fact that no one who had syphilis was ever able to talk about it. To call a respectable person syphilitic was unthinkable. To share that you were someone with syphilis with anyone but your closest intimates was similarly unthinkable. Perhaps you wouldn't even wish to share the diagnosis even with your closest intimates.

The same Upton Sinclair novel in which the doctor describes the woman whose lips have rotted away revolves around a young man named George who, after cheating on his fiancée, discovers he has syphilis. Unable to break off the engagement without ruining their reputation, he marries her, never tells her he has syphilis, and infects her. She in turn infects their newborn child. The newborn then infects the family's wet nurse. The compounding repercussions of George's secret seem incredibly realistic.

When George first sees the red sore that he, correctly, identifies as a sign that he is a syphilitic, he confides in a friend. This exchange follows:

> The friend was willing to talk. It was a vile disease, he said; but one was foolish to bother about it, because it was so rare. There were other diseases which fellows got, which nearly every fellow had, and to which none of them paid any attention. But one seldom met anyone who had the red plague that George dreaded.
>
> "And yet," he added, "according to the books, it isn't so uncommon. I suppose the truth is that people hide it. A chap naturally wouldn't tell, when he knew it would damn him for life."

George had a sick sensation inside of him. "Is it as bad as that?" he asked.

"Of course," said the other. "Should you want to have anything to do with a person who had it? Should you be willing to room with him or travel with him? You wouldn't even want to shake hands with him!"

Terror of and reluctance to associate with known syphilitics, especially if you were unsure of exactly how the disease spread, is an understandable response. And it was difficult to educate people on something they *did not want to hear about.* People barely even referred to syphilis by name; they often called it a "rare blood disease." As late as 1906, when *Ladies' Home Journal* published a series of articles about STDs including a discussion of syphilis, it lost seventy-five thousand subscribers.[20]

You might marvel that anyone could hide a disease that resulted in their nose rotting off their face. It's possible, though. My wonderful agent tells a story of how her great-grandfather had a wooden nosepiece that he wore when he had to go into town. His family claimed his nose had rotted away because it was always being flicked by cows' tails. My agent now realizes that a cover-up might have been in play.

Hiding the disease led to disastrous outcomes. That began to become clear to people during the divorce case between Lord Colin Campbell and his wife in 1886. Lady Campbell, née Gertrude Blood, agreed to marry Lord Colin after a three-day romance in Scotland when she was age twenty-two. It seemed great! Campbell was rich, Lady Gertrude was poor, and they . . . liked each other as much as you can after three days. The only problem was that Lord Colin Campbell had syphilis. They didn't consummate their marriage right away (Lord Campbell was operating on the assumption that the symptoms would go away, and they'd be able to consummate their union more safely), but according to the *Times*: "In October of 1881, after remaining in London, the parties went to Bournemouth and there, the marriage not having been then consummated, Lord Colin passed a slip of paper to his wife, purporting to contain an extract from a doctor's letter, which said that if they now occupied the same room it would be beneficial to Lord Colin. They went to Inverary later in October, and there, for the first time, intercourse took place."[21]

It may well have been beneficial to Lord Campbell, but not Lady Campbell. She was infected with syphilis within months. By 1883 she obtained a degree of separation, claiming "cruelty"— the cruelty being that he gave her syphilis. You cannot imagine how genuinely shocked people were by this news at the trial. According to the biography *Love Well the Hour: The Life of Lady Colin Campbell (1857–1911)* by Anne Jordan, Gertrude's lawyer, Sir Charles Russell, "exposed what he attested was the true nature of Colin's illness—syphilis. Most of the newspapers ignored it, skirted the issue, or like *The Times* indicated that the coverage would be 'utterly unfit for the columns of a newspaper.'"[22] The press struggled to report accurately on the trial. The *Evening News* was charged with "obscene libel" by the National Vigilance Association for putting the word *syphilis* in print. The public, despite gobbling up the details about the trial—the *Evening News's* circulation had doubled—were *furious* that anyone had written about the disease at all.

Look. If you have ever read *Harry Potter*, you know that being so afraid of something that you cannot speak its name only makes that thing more terrifying.

The judge didn't grant Lord and Lady Campbell a divorce, but he did seem to favor Lady Campbell, asking, "Do you think Lord Colin Campbell's attempt to treat his wife as a common prostitute was anything short of an outrage?"[23]

Yes, it was outrageous! Lord Colin Campbell should have been more candid about the nature of his disease, especially since Lady Campbell *couldn't read or learn about it anywhere.*

However, continually reinforcing the concept that only monsters or common prostitutes contracted the disease did not make people *more* likely to talk about having syphilis. It would be great even today if people could talk about STDs without hissing "sinner" at the people who have the mere misfortune of contracting them.

The silence around the nature of syphilis continued for many years. It laid the groundwork that made the horrific Tuskegee Syphilis Study possible. During that shameful experiment the effects of untreated syphilis on six hundred rural African American men were studied. They were never told they had the disease. The experiment would last for forty years from 1932 to 1972. Participants were never told that as of 1947 it was known that pencillan would cure their disease. (Studies of this sort now, fortunately, require *informed consent* by participants.) The Tuskegee Study was utterly diabolical, but it was made possible because a culture of ignorance surrounding syphilis was embraced. This is the kind of thing that happens when you have a disease that most of the population is kept entirely in the dark about or views with only vague, abstract terror. This is what happens when silence and shaming campaigns are considered acceptable responses to diseases.

Which is why I think the hero of this story is not only the inventor of penicillin. (The inventor of penicillin, which cures syphilis, is Alexander Fleming. He is great. So is the lesser-known Howard Florey. *Alexander Fleming: The Man and the Myth* by Gwyn Macfarlane is a very good biography in which you can read and learn more about both of them.) My favorite hero can be found in a reference in an 1818 edition of *Blackwood's Edinburgh Magazine*, which described a unique London club called the "No Nose'd Club." The author writes: "A certain whimsical gentleman having taken a fancy to see a large party of noseless persons invited every one he met to dine on a certain day at a tavern, where he formed them all into a brotherhood bearing the above name." The man, who is referred to as Mr. Crumpton, apparently gathered a large group of noseless, syphilitic people. Surely, most of them were unused to seeing others suffering from the some disease they were. "As the number increased the surprise grew the greater among all that were present who stared at one another with such unaccustomed bashfulness and confused oddness as if every sinner beheld their own iniquities in the faces of their companions."[24]

Let's skim over the fact that they're called sinners and marvel instead at what it must have been like to finally connect with other people who shared their affliction. To be able to *talk* to others about a disease that most people were afraid to name. If they were shocked, that reaction seems understandable; most of them would have spent much of their time covering up their noselessness as best they could. According to the article, the men got along and began making jokes almost immediately: " 'If we should fall together by the ears how long might we all fight before we should have bloody noses?' 'Ads flesh,' says another, 'now you talk of noses I have been looking this half hour to find one in the company.' 'God be praised,' says a third, 'though we have no noses we have every one a mouth and that by spreading of the table seems at present to be the most useful member.' "[25]

They sound like a fun bunch. They have no noses, but they still have their senses of humor! My favorite people are those who can make jokes when most of us would despair. And look, this may be the first record of people with syphilis being portrayed in a way that doesn't make them seem like they are somehow inhuman—either as genius creative monsters or as just plain ogres. The fact that the sufferers are depicted as real people was a big step, even if the disease's actual name is never referenced in the article.

Shaming people for contracting a disease that we don't have a cure for is still common today. In part we want to believe that those people are not like us. We like to believe that people somehow brought diseases on themselves, but diseases are mindless and do not judiciously pick the worst people in the world to murder. The more we distance ourselves from diseases and their victims, the harder it becomes to educate people about prevention or raise the funds for a cure (because why would you want to cure something only monstrous people get?). Portraying the afflicted in a way that acknowledges their suffering but also shows them to be brave and humorous and able to joke makes them seem like any one of us.

Sadly, according to the article, the founder of the No Nose'd Club died after a year—likely of syphilis—and the "flat faced community were unhappily dissolved." In the final meeting, the following poem was recited in honor of the founder:

> Mourn for the loss of such a friend
> Whose lofty Nose
> no humble snout disdained
> But tho of Roman height could stoop so low
> As to sooth those who ne'er a Nose shew
> Ah sure no noseless club could ever find
> One single Nose so bountiful and kind
> But now alas! He's sunk into the deep
> Where neither kings nor slaves a Nose shall keep
> But where proud Beauties strutting Beaux and all
> Must soon into the noseless fashion fall
> Thither your friend in complaisance is gone
> To have his Nose, like yours, reduced to none.[26]

That's a much more enjoyable poem than the one praising syphilis we read earlier.

Diseases don't ruin lives just because they rot off noses. They destroy people if the rest of society isolates them and treats them as undeserving of help and respect. In the best cases, like Strasbourg during the dancing plague, communities come together to care for their weakest members. In other cases, outside supporters might take up the cause of these people as their own. But more often, the ill are forced to look to others like themselves to find strength. Those describing the No Nose'd Club regarded it as a humorous—and maybe even bizarre—novelty, but the formation of this group helped lay the groundwork for associations for those suffering from diseases ranging from alcoholism to AIDS.

The members of Mr. Crumpton's club were—at least while they were together—liberated from shame about their disease. That is a great thing because shame is one of the enemies in the war on diseases. Shaming people cures nothing. Living in a state of silence cures nothing. It only means that more people are afraid to talk about their ailments. That means that they're at a disadvantage, because they can't protect themselves against things they barely know about. When we raise our voices, whether it's in a small group, like Mr. Crumpton's, or in a larger number, we say that we will not allow ourselves to be killed. We say that we don't deserve to suffer, even if hypocrites in society believe we do. And once society begins to hear those voices, it will, we hope, begin to work harder to find a cure.

Tuberculosis

Dying of tuberculosis. The earth is suffocating . . . Swear to make them cut me open, so that I won't be buried alive.

—Frédéric Chopin

Throughout history, as we've seen with syphilis, people have wanted to glamorize certain diseases. They really shouldn't. Diseases are not lovely under any circumstances. Pretending they are is about as effective as trying to paint a pretty face on a death mask. Applying some lipstick to a skull doesn't turn it into Jennifer Lawrence. Diseases are the most fundamental enemy of the human race, and we must be at constant war against them.

Here are some things that diseases don't make people:

- Cool
- Poetic
- Sexy
- Classy
- Genius

Here is one thing they do make people:

• Dead

If only this was understood by the numerous people in the nineteenth century who thought that tuberculosis was just *So. Damn. Glamorous.*

Tuberculosis—which was often called consumption—is a bacterial disease. It is very contagious. The bacterium is spread by droplets whenever sufferers cough or sneeze (or sing or laugh, for that matter). Those droplets are then inhaled by others. In some people, the bacterium remains latent for years. In others, it goes into remission. And in the most serious cases the bacterium settles in the lungs, where it eventually destroys their tissue. Symptoms include chest pain, coughing, severe weight loss, and that spitting-blood-into-a-handkerchief thing (the technical name for that is bloody sputum) you are definitely familiar with if you have seen the movie *Moulin Rouge* (2001).[1]

In many literary works from the nineteenth century, consumption is the death of choice for beautiful angelic women. Their fictional final moments almost always have them dying peacefully and looking great as they slip away. For instance, in Harriet Beecher Stowe's *Uncle Tom's Cabin*, published in 1852:

> It soon became quite plain to everybody that Eva was very ill indeed. She never ran about and played now, but spent most of the day lying on the sofa in her own pretty room.
>
> Everyone loved her, and tried to do things for her. Even naughty little Topsy used to bring her flowers, and try to be good for her sake . . .
>
> One day Eva made her aunt cut off a lot of her beautiful hair. Then she called all the slaves together, said good-bye to them, and gave them each a curl of her hair as a keepsake.

They all cried very much and said they would never forget
her, and would try to be good for her sake . . . in the morning
little Eva lay on her bed, cold and white, with closed eyes and
folded hands.[2]

In his lesser-known short story *Metzengerstein*, published in
1832, Edgar Allan Poe wrote: "The beautiful Lady Mary! How
could she die?—and of consumption! But it is a path I have
prayed to follow. I would wish all I love to perish of that gentle
disease. How glorious! to depart in the hey-day of the young
blood—the heart of all passion—the imagination all fire—amid
the remembrances of happier days—in the fall of the year—and
so be buried up forever in the gorgeous autumnal leaves!"[3] You
can certainly argue that Poe was enamored with death in general, but Victor Hugo wasn't. His work didn't usually fetishize
death. And yet here is his description of Fantine on her deathbed in *Les Misérables* (1862):

She was asleep. Her breath issued from her breast with that
tragic sound which is peculiar to those maladies, and which
breaks the hearts of mothers when they are watching
through the night beside their sleeping child who is condemned to death. But this painful respiration hardly troubled
a sort of ineffable serenity which overspread her countenance,
and which transfigured her in her sleep. Her pallor had
become whiteness; her cheeks were crimson; her long golden
lashes, the only beauty of her youth and her virginity which
remained to her, palpitated, though they remained closed and
drooping. Her whole person was trembling with an inde-
scribable unfolding of wings, all ready to open wide and bear
her away, which could be felt as they rustled, though they
could not be seen. To see her thus, one would never have
dreamed that she was an invalid whose life was almost

despaired of. She resembled rather something on the point of soaring away than something on the point of dying.[4]

Something soaring *like an angel*.

And this glamorous tuberculosis trope was not confined to novels. Verdi's opera *La Traviata* (inspired by Alexandre Dumas's *La Dame Aux Camelias*, published in 1848) was first staged in 1853. The story revolves around the tragic but decadent life of the courtesan Violetta. She is perhaps history's most famous consumptive and was at least part of the inspiration for Nicole Kidman's character in *Moulin Rouge*. Violetta dies singing: "The spasms of pain are ceasing / In me . . . is born / I am moved by an unaccustomed strength! / Oh! But I . . . oh! / I'm returning to life! / Oh, joy!" Her last note is a high B-flat, which no one with tuberculosis would ever be able to hit, partly because it would require too much lung expansion, and partly because tuberculosis often resulted in hoarseness owing to tubercular laryngitis.[5] Oh well. It's a good song.

Owing in part to these euphemistic portrayals, during the nineteenth century people were not especially afraid of tuberculosis. The general thought was that, okay, you die, but it's a really easy death and you're all pale and sexy like an angel or a character in a Tim Burton movie.

You know who didn't feel this way? The men and women who actually had tuberculosis. The actress Elisa Rachel Félix would have begged to differ with anyone who thought she looked *amazing* when she was sick with consumption in 1855. She claimed: "You who knew Rachel in the brilliance of her splendor and the riot of her glory, who have so often heard the theater ring with her triumphs—you would not believe that the gaunt spectre which now drags itself wearily over the world is— Rachel." She died of suffocation in 1858 while (trying) to cry out for her deceased sister.[6]

It wasn't just women with tuberculosis who were thought of as dying of a painless but beautiful malady. The poet Byron once told a friend, "I should like, I think, to die of consumption; because then the women would all say, 'See the poor Byron—how interesting he looks in dying!'"[7] The romantic poet John Keats was the poster boy for dying of "that gentle disease." Percy Bysshe Shelley claimed that Keats contracted the disease because "the savage criticism of his [poem] *Endymion* produced the most violent effect on his susceptible mind. The agitation thus originated ended in the rupture of a blood vessel in the lungs."[8]

You can be upset, but I don't think you can die from a bad review. This is the only time when I have seen literary critics called actual murderers, but Shelley said it, so think about the power you wield the next time you log on to Goodreads.

When Keats was suffering the symptoms of maybe-bad-review-induced tuberculosis during his visit to Rome in 1820, he was treated by Dr. James Clark, who seemingly did not think things were all that dire. Upon learning that Keats had been put in a separate ward in a Roman hospital with other consumptives due to the risk of contagion, Dr. Clark sniffed that this arrangement was "maintained by the vulgar," and that it originated from "the old and almost obsolete opinion of the contagious nature of this disease."[9] We will put aside the fact that referring to people maintaining a hospital as "vulgar" makes him sound like a pretentious ass.

Let's focus instead on the fact that tuberculosis is in fact *extremely* contagious. The Roman hospitals were using sensible protocols. Dr. Clark would have been even more unimpressed if he had been to Spain, where the populace was even more vigilant in their attempts to prevent the spread of the disease. In that country not only did consumptives have to be reported and moved to a hospital immediately; following their deaths even their houses were declared virtually uninhabitable.

But Dr. Clark had none of these quaint concerns. When he

was trying to treat Keats, he put him on a diet of anchovies and bread. He claimed that the disease "seems seated in his stomach."[10] He was not alone in thinking that various foods might cure consumption. Daniel Whitney wrote in *The Family Physician, and Guide to Health* (1833) that "Dr. Mudge cured himself by keeping constantly open an issue between his shoulders of fifty peas, and by using at the same time a milk and vegetable diet."[11] The peas, which were presumably intended to agitate the skin and produce a discharge, seem to be a weird anomaly, but the milk and vegetable diet likely stemmed from the theories proffered by Dr. Edward Barry in his *Treatise on the Consumption of Lungs* (1726). Dr. Barry, who was one of the most acclaimed physicians of the time, claimed that British people of "a better sort" contracted tuberculosis because they tended to imbibe liquor and eat a lot of meat. He deduced they could therefore combat the disease through a diet of milk and vegetables.[12]

Eating vegetables is never a bad idea. Neither is drinking milk instead of brandy or claret or whatever else eighteenth-century British aristocrats were downing. If you want to keep a bunch of uncomfortable peas between your shoulders—okay, free to be you and me. However, this nutritional regime would not cure you. It certainly didn't save Keats, and the bloodletting that was additionally prescribed probably hastened his decline. He died at age twenty-six. His life was so brief that he wished for his tombstone simply to read "Here lies one whose life was writ in water." Meanwhile, Dr. Clark went on to become Physician-in-Ordinary to Queen Victoria and lived out his life in a magnificent estate, which seems unfair.

Anchovies aside, Keats's death is often remembered as something peaceful and romantic and dreamy. That's partly due to his writing poems like "Ode to a Nightingale" that opine:

> Darkling I listen; and, for many a time
> I have been half in love with easeful Death,

Call'd him soft names in many a mused rhyme,
To take into the air my quiet breath;
Now more than ever seems it rich to die,
To cease upon the midnight with no pain

Blame for this faulty angelic remembrance also lies with Keats's good friend Joseph Severn, who was at the poet's deathbed. Severn recalled Keats's death in later years as a "good death," toeing the whole "consumption is a beautiful way to go" party line.

However, Severn's private letters from the time when Keats was dying tell a very different story. He wrote to his friend Charles Brown on December 17, 1820, about a month before Keats died:

> Five times the blood has come up in coughing, in large quantities [around two cups' worth] generally in the morning, and nearly the whole time his saliva has been mixed with it. But this is the lesser evil when compared with his Stomach. Not a single thing will digest. The torture he suffers all and every night and best part of the day is dreadful in the extreme. The distended stomach keeps him in perpetual hunger or craving, and this is augmented by the little nourishment he takes to keep down the blood. Then his mind is worse than all—despair in every shape. His imagination and memory present every image in horror, so strong that morning and night I tremble for his intellect.[13]

That is what death from tuberculosis was like. It's not cool and peaceful. There's no such thing as a good death but especially not that one. Keats's death sounds like something from a Lovecraft story.

So how did a disease that is *so* gruesome and bloody gain this reputation for turning sufferers into beautiful angels?

Tuberculosis was, even early on, associated with attractiveness. The first-century physician Aretaeus of Cappadocia described the typical sufferer as having a "nose sharp, slender; cheeks prominent and red; eyes hollow, brilliant and glittering."[14] Admittedly, big-eyed and skinny with rosy cheeks is a description that sounds a lot like today's supermodels.

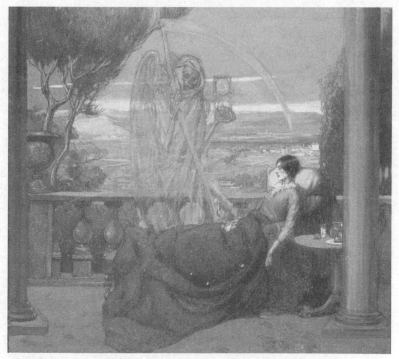

So . . . do you have a boyfriend?

The association of consumption and beauty endured for thousands of years. In 1726, in the aforementioned treatise on the *Consumption of the Lungs*, Dr. Barry wrote that people suffering from tuberculosis generally physically presented:

> [a] long Neck, Scapulae prominent like wings, Thorax compressed, and narrow, a clear florid Complexion, the Cheeks and lips painted with the purest red, the Caruncle [small

piece of flesh] in the Corner of the Eye, from its intense Colour, appears like Coral; and all the vessels are so fine, as to appear almost diaphanous: Such Persons are likewise most frequently remarkable for a Vivacity of Mind.[15]

And in 1833 Daniel H. Whitney still claimed that you could recognize a consumptive by "clean fair skin, bright eyes, white teeth, delicate rosy complexion, sanguine temperament, great sensibility, thick lips."[16]

This is a good moment to point out that *tuberculosis doesn't make your neck long*. As late as the nineteenth century, the poet and physician Tomas Lovell Beddoes goes on about the long, lovely necks of consumptives.[17] I (not a doctor) can attribute the other physical descriptions to the extreme weight loss that accompanies tuberculosis—because your body has to expend more energy keeping you alive—as well as being flushed with fever, but the idea that the disease either produces a long neck or is due to one is just incorrect. If you were thinking consumption would turn you into a Modigliani model, it won't.

It is also worth pointing out that a bacterial disease doesn't make you smarter or more possessed of a "Vivacity of Mind."

Not only were those suffering from tuberculosis supposedly beautiful and brilliant; according to Christian tradition they were also godly and good. That belief was mostly due to the association of plumpness with worldly appetites of many kinds. If you were as bony as someone with consumption, you must have been depriving yourself in this world to feast with Jesus in the next.[18]

You will be hard-pressed to find any portrayal where consumptives aren't *gorgeous*—beautiful, otherworldly, and quite sexy. Sexy because, as Hippocrates noted in the fifth century, consumption tended to attack young people, chiefly between the ages of eighteen and thirty-five.[19]

Given the age and perceived attractiveness of the sufferers, in the seventeenth century tuberculosis was thought to be a disease caused by lovesickness. Gideon Harvey, the physician to King Charles II of England, was certain that consumption was linked to love. In *Of an Amorous Consumption*, he explains that "when Maids do suddenly grow thin-jawed and hollow-eyed, they are certainly in Love."[20] Weight loss, a lack of appetite, and eye glitter could be caused by some unrequited passion. They just weren't in the cases of people who were actually ill with tuberculosis. The theory went further. If sadness from a lack of love caused the disease, it could be *cured* by love. That was utterly untrue, but the idea of dying from lovesickness is more palatable than the idea of dying from rotting lungs. Unfortunately, this reasoning meant that a terrifying, deadly disease was reduced to something seen as delightful and ladylike.

By the late eighteenth century—and certainly the turn of the nineteenth—even women who did not have consumption wanted to *look* as though they did. Of course, to be concerned about fashionable appearances you had to have money and time to spare. Medical attention and information about consumption were accordingly targeted directly to a "well-bred" audience. In John Armstrong's *Art of Preserving Health* (1744), he directs his thoughts on tuberculosis to "ye finer souls / Form'd to soft luxury."[21] At the turn of the nineteenth century, Beddoes complained of boarding schools that had "greatly contributed to multiply the genteel, linear, consumptive make, now or lately so much in request." The nineteenth-century doctor Thomas Trotter likewise lamented: "So unnatural and perverted are fashionable opinions on this subject, that a blooming complexion is thought to indicate low life and vulgarity in breeding. What a false standard for beauty: to prefer a sickly sallow hue of the countenance to the roses of health!"[22] Women began covering themselves in whitening powder during this period—the idea of a suntan to show health and an outdoorsy spirit wouldn't be popular until the twentieth century.[23]

All of these conceptions about the disease being for the well-born were incorrect. Of course tuberculosis could affect any member of society regardless of their social rank. Between 1829 and 1845, 10 to 13 percent of white prisoners in large cities on the East Coast of the United States died of tuberculosis; the rate was even higher among black prisoners.[24] Overcrowded housing conditions in the nineteenth century meant that tuberculosis was prevalent among the poor, so much so that Marx and Engels later labeled the disease a "necessary condition to the existence of capital."[25] In 1815 the physician Thomas Young claimed that it was "a disease so frequent as to carry off prematurely about one-fourth part of the inhabitants of Europe."[26] Indeed, about 4 million people were thought to have died from consumption in England and Wales alone between 1851 and 1910.[27]

The fact that even today tuberculosis is often associated with dying aristocrats is probably because there was a whole lifestyle marketed to well-heeled sufferers. Inducements to visit the warm climate of the Mediterranean promised that it was "the last ditch of the consumptive."[28] Every seaside village seemed to claim that its salt water could cure the disease. And then there was the big-city opera cure. In *The White Plague: Tuberculosis, Man and Society*, Jean and René Dubos explain: "Nice was the most fashionable rendezvous for those who tried to dodge death every winter by escaping from northern frosts. At the Opera House, performances of the 'cooing, phthisical' music of the Romantic Era nightly attracted throngs of corpselike consumptives. The young women were smartly dressed and lavishly jeweled, but so pale beneath their curls that their faces appeared to be powdered with 'scrapings' of bones."[29] Jewels! Gowns! Romantic music! It all sounds so glamorous! No wonder the musician character in Henri Murger's 1851 *Scènes de la Vie de Bohème* gripes, "I would be famous as the sun if I had a black suit, wore long hair and one of my lungs was diseased."

If the seashore or the opera didn't strike your fancy, there were many mountain sanatoriums for those who could afford them, like the one depicted by Thomas Mann in *The Magic Mountain* (1924). They were places where wealthy consumptives could spend their days enjoying rest cures while taking, at least if Mann's depiction is to be believed, a great deal of pleasure in their elite diseased status. Their popularity originated with the German physician Hermann Brehmer's initially unpopular theory that tuberculosis could be cured by plenty of rest in a high altitude. At these sanatoriums "guests" would rest on open, airy porches, eat decadent meals (Brehmer and his colleagues believed in feeding consumptives more than milk and vegetables), and go for walks in nature. And if you felt you needed more stimulation than a mountain sanatorium could provide, the poet Sidney Lanier proposed, in what is certainly the most bizarre suggestion I have found, that consumptives could move to the wonderful climate of Florida and begin hunting alligators, so as to sell the animals' teeth at a handsome price from four to ten dollars a pound. He was not joking.[30]

The idea of becoming a professional alligator hunter when you can scarcely breathe sounds dicey. Lanier's plan aside, sleeping for most of the day, traipsing to the opera in jewels, and traveling to Nice or the Alps "for your health" sounds like fun to me. Being constantly told you are beautiful/handsome and sensitive like an angel sounds even more enjoyable. The only part of this lifestyle that sounds terrible is the "dying in agony" part, which is—always—glossed over. Beddoes claimed he was facing an uphill battle in convincing the "ghostly beauties of court and city that to be robust and in 'rude' or vulgar health is not a 'curse.'"[31]

It's easy, given all of the associations regarding wealth and beauty, to forget that tuberculosis is caused by bacteria. It doesn't have a brain. It doesn't choose. It preys on absolutely anyone it comes into contact with, beautiful or ugly, rich or poor, smart or street smart, maybe—not book smart.

Bacteria don't infect people based on their personality traits or income. However, given the glamor and status associated with the disease, Beddoes came to the conclusion that women were deliberately contracting consumption to look more chic.

Tragically, the fetishization of this sickly physical ideal did indeed lead some women who were naturally healthy to become sickly, even if they did not contract consumption itself. The unfortunate death of poor Lizzie Siddal was an example where glamorizing a tubercular aesthetic turned deadly. In addition to being a poet and painter herself, Siddal was perhaps the most famous artist's model and muse of the Pre-Raphaelite era. You would probably recognize her from paintings like John Everett Millais's *Ophelia* and Dante Gabriel Rossetti's *Beata Beatrix*. She was known for her slimness and pallor, her long red hair, and for looking as if she was dying of tuberculosis. It was generally believed at the time that she had the disease; indeed, the scholar Katherine Byrne explained that "her attractiveness was inseparable from her perceived consumptive state."[32]

Here's the thing: she probably didn't have tuberculosis. Today, it seems more likely that she was suffering from anorexia (she wrote letters to her lover Rossetti telling him that she had not eaten for weeks) and a serious addiction to opiates.[33] Ideally—ideally!—good health would not be seen as a vulgar curse, and someone would have said, "Hey, Lizzie, you look very sick; let's see if we can find a way to address this issue because it might have to do with you not eating for weeks on end and also your laudanum habit. I know we are in the Victorian age, and accordingly everything is awful, and mothers are giving their infants laudanum in an ill-advised attempt to soothe them, so *babies* are getting addicted. Seriously, it is amazing how many drugs everyone is doing right now, everyone is just drugged to the gills, but still, Lizzie. Still."

That is just how we would say it. We are very good at confronting problems head-on. We would take Lizzie back to the future with us in our time machine. We would have to take Lizzie to a time when disordered eating and drug addiction aren't problems for models and other women pressured to fit society's definition of beauty, so . . . oh.

As is, tragically, still the case today when some women engage in destructive behaviors, people didn't want to help Lizzie so much as they wanted to praise how fashionable and skinny she looked. When the painter Ford Madox Brown visited her, he enthused, "Miss Siddal—looking thinner and more deathlike and more beautiful and more ragged than ever."[34] (*Deathlike* and *beautiful* went together so easily.)

In *Tuberculosis and the Victorian Literary Imagination* Katherine Byrne writes, "It seems that [Siddal's] desirability lay in her fragility and that she was special because she always seemed hovering on the verge of death, and looked as though she was not quite of this world."[35] This poor depressed, drug addicted, possibly anorexic woman.

Elizabeth Siddal died horribly of a laudanum overdose in what may have been a suicide. She was age thirty-two.

Fortunately, ideals about beauty can change. As the years went on, romantic depictions of tuberculosis and the lives of those suffering from it gave way to more realistic descriptions. In 1877 when Tolstoy published *Anna Karenina*, he presented a very different vision of what someone dying of tuberculosis looks like from those pretty pictures of Fantine or Violetta. This one bears a closer resemblance to Severn's description of Keats's death, likely because Tolstoy based the scene on his brothers' actual deaths from tuberculosis in 1856 and 1860.

[Nikolai's brother] had expected to find the physical signs of the approach of death more marked—greater weakness, greater emaciation, but still almost the same condition of things. He had expected himself to feel the same distress at the loss of the brother he loved and the same horror in face of death as he had felt then, only in a greater degree. And he had prepared himself for this; but he found something utterly different.

In a little dirty room with the painted panels of its walls filthy with spittle, and conversation audible through the thin partition from the next room, in a stifling atmosphere saturated with impurities, on a bedstead moved away from the wall, there lay covered with a quilt, a body. One arm of this body was above the quilt, and the wrist, huge as a rake-handle, was attached, inconceivably it seemed, to the thin, long bone of the arm smooth from the beginning to the middle. The head lay sideways on the pillow. Levin could see the scanty locks wet with sweat on the temples and tense, transparent-looking forehead . . . Only at rare moments, when the opium gave him an instant's relief from the never-ceasing pain, he would sometimes, half asleep, utter what was ever more intense in his heart than in all the others: "Oh, if it were only the end!" or: "When will it be over?" His sufferings, steadily growing more intense, did their work and prepared him for death. There was no position in which he was not in pain, there was not a minute in which he was unconscious of it, not a limb, not a part of his body that did not ache and cause him agony.[36]

Good for Tolstoy for making death from tuberculosis sound terrible. When diseases sound frightful, people stop thinking they are a minor ailment alleviated by eating anchovies or bathing in salt water or falling in love.

As the nineteenth century neared its close, it was becoming clear that at least some people were fed up with the whole "let's just have people eat alternative foods and go on vacation" attempts to treat the disease. Jacques Offenbach's opera *The Tales of Hoffmann* (1881) pokes fun at medical charlatans through the character of Dr. Miracle, whose inept methods inadvertently kill the lovely heroine Antonia in the second act. The absurdities of the doctor's treatments would have been recognizable to many in the audience.

Now, were these new artistic characterizations of the disease anywhere near as popular as the depictions of women dying like gorgeous angels? No, of course not! Many people—though presumably not you, because you saw this disease-riddled book and said, "That is a book for me!"—don't like hearing about the more gruesome aspects of life. In general people want to read about happy stuff and to feel good and to look at puppies wearing party hats.

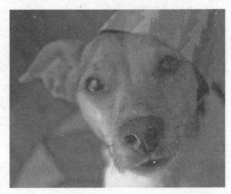

Who's a healthy boy?!

Fortunately, there are individuals who can create art that is so good that it can't help but educate people about life's gritty realities. Those tales generally cleverly offset bad news with more appealing aspects. Nobody reads *Anna Karenina* because they want to see how Nikolai dies. They read it because they hate trains. Or because they love enduring tales of passion. Either/or. Nobody goes to *The Tales of Hoffmann* because they are into medical quackery of the nineteenth century. I think most people go for the music and costumes. But Tolstoy and Offenbach still managed to insert in their works enlightening messages about the realities of a terrible disease.

God bless anyone whose work holds up a mirror to the world.

The romantic appeal of the disease dissipated further in 1882 when the German bacteriologist Robert Koch identified the bacilli that caused consumption by using a microscope and a stained sample (which was extremely cutting-edge technology at the time). He also determined how tuberculosis spread from one person to the next, proving it was not caused by having a lot of feelings, being rich, or being beautiful.[37]

In his writings, known for their realism, the American author Upton Sinclair began associating the disease with working-class people, not "finer souls, form'd to soft luxury."[38] The opera *La Bohème* (1895) also associated the disease with poor people. Admittedly, poor creative people, but poor nonetheless. It also didn't portray it as a disease that went hand in hand with love and a glamorous life on earth. The beautiful Mimi's consumption causes her to be abandoned by her lover, as he sings, "Amo Mimi, ma ho paura" (I love Mimi, but I'm afraid).

As tuberculosis came to be regarded less as an ailment specific to the stylish elite and more (correctly) as a huge public health problem, clinics like the Victoria Dispensary for Consumption and Diseases of the Chest began opening. The French declared "War on Tuberculosis," and in 1886 the Conseil d'Hygiène et de Salubrité voted to outlaw public spitting. By 1909 the radical Thaddeus Browne was writing poetry about consumption as a disease that was "malignant, repellent, appalling."[39] People raced to develop vaccine therapies, and any notions about how captivating consumption was faded in the light of medical knowledge.

By 1921 the Bacille Calmette-Guérin vaccine, which is still used today, was developed. It is currently administered to around 100 million children worldwide. In areas where tuberculosis is still prevalent, it is recommended that children receive the vaccine as soon as possible after birth. In the event that someone contracts tuberculosis, there are now ten antibiotics approved by the FDA to treat the disease over a course of six to nine months.[40]

The good news is that we now know tuberculosis isn't a cool blessing. We don't look at a woman with consumption and think, *Oh, man, she is withered like a ghost and spitting blood; I want her to be my Victorian bride.* The fact that we are at least slightly less inclined to wholeheartedly glamorize conditions that kill people is a step forward for humans. The downside is that we often don't think about those suffering from tuberculosis at all. The disease is still around, it's still contagious, and despite the fact that the vaccine costs approximately sixteen cents to produce, and $3.13 to buy, tuberculosis continues to ravage periphery countries.[41]

Millions of people worldwide die from tuberculosis every year—*and it's totally treatable.* This is a disease we can eradicate in our lifetime. Because we are modern people! We know that diseases aren't friendly, they aren't cool, and they're not even a good excuse to become an alligator hunter. So you have two options in fighting the good fight against a universal enemy. Either you can create great art that illustrates the plight of people dying from tuberculosis, as Tolstoy did, or you can donate $1.30 (for the 1.3 million people who die of the disease each year) to any of the worthy organizations that fight tuberculosis. If you're going with the latter option, I recommend the Stop TB Partnership, which is endorsed by the United Nations Foundation and does amazing work. If you choose the former, I hear wine helps some people write books.

Cholera

*His examination revealed that he had
no fever, no pain anywhere, and that
his only concrete feeling was an
urgent desire to die. All that was
needed was shrewd questioning . . .
to conclude once again that the
symptoms of love were the same
as those of cholera.*

—GABRIEL GARCÍA MÁRQUEZ

Once people think they understand how something works, it takes a veritable force of nature to convince them differently. Seriously. Try it. Try to change someone's mind about one fact or situation or process they believe they understand fully. You can use as much data as you want. You can make diagrams. You can write a song and put on a damn musical. They will not believe you—because their fourth-grade teacher told them something different, and they are certain they *already know how it works*.

Remember how much it upset people when we were told that Pluto wasn't a planet anymore? I'm still mad about that. The only thing I knew for sure about space was "the order of all the planets" (My Very Educated Mother Just Served Us Nine Pizzas), and then that one bit of knowledge was ripped away from me. What mnemonic do kids even use now? I'm aware there are reasons Pluto was demoted, but in my heart, I do not care what Neil deGrasse Tyson says. (Even though I know in my mind he's right, in my heart, I feel he's wrong.)

So, on that note, remember how during the bubonic plague everyone thought that the disease might be caused by foul, smelly air? The doctors wore cool bird masks filled with cloves and potpourri, which they believed would stop them from catching the disease. And remember how we all laughed and collectively said, "That's dumb!" because we know diseases aren't caused by bad smells in the air? Well, the belief that diseases stemmed from bad smells lasted longer than you could possibly imagine. Five hundred more years. It lingered—like the stench of a dead fish—all the way into the 1850s. In 1844 Professor H. Booth even went so far as to claim in the journal of architecture the *Builder* that "from inhaling the odour of beef the butcher's wife obtains her obesity."[1]

This seems like an unfair stereotype about butchers' wives.

In 1846 the social reformer Edwin Chadwick gave a speech before British parliament claiming: "All smell is, if it be intense, immediate acute disease; and eventually we may say that, by depressing the system and rendering it susceptible to the action of other causes, all smell is disease."[2] Even the celebrated nurse Florence Nightingale believed that measles, scarlet fever, and smallpox were caused by bad odors.

This theory led to some bizarre ideas. For instance, Chadwick thought that tall structures like the Eiffel Tower could be used to allow people to collect clean, good-smelling air from the top levels, which would then be distributed, "warmed and fresh," to people below.[3] I am fascinated by the mechanics of how Chadwick thought this could be done. I don't know how he was going to effectively transport air from the highest point of the Eiffel Tower. A basket? Maybe jars. I guess jars would be best. I imagine he was going to have hundreds of people climb

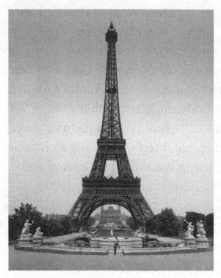

Definitely a super practical structure

to the top of the Eiffel Tower with jars, collect fresh air, and then transport it to ground level, where they'd heat it like a loaf of bread and share it with everyone. It seems like an unworkable idea, but a fun image to have in your head when you visit the Eiffel Tower.

The conviction that bad smells caused disease had some upsides in London. It resulted in a massive effort to clean up the streets and houses, which were filled with filth, which was generally the source of noxious odors. Chadwick was quoted in the *Times* in 1849 saying that the effort should apply first to the "purification of the dwelling house, next of the street and lastly of the river."[4] The Nuisances Removal and Diseases Prevention Act of 1846 seemed to proceed in accordance with the order Chadwick later suggested.

Any movement toward sanitization is usually also a step forward in combatting disease. London during the mid-nineteenth century was wildly overcrowded. Its population of 2.5 million made it the largest city in the world at that time. (That's roughly the size of Chicago today.) One census described a single room where five families were living, each in their own area. They claimed they were doing well with four families (and four corners) until someone took in a lodger in the middle. And then there was the livestock that people kept inside their houses. We're not talking about livestock in the sense of "a few people had some chickens." We're talking cows in the attics. They'd be levered up by pulley and kept in the attic as long as they had milk to give. (If I had such a cow, I would name her Bertha Mason.) It wasn't always even one or two cows; there might be as many as thirty cows in what were known as "cow houses."[5] One man kept twenty-seven dogs in his one-room apartment! Another woman down the street had seventeen cats, dogs, and rabbits.

Meanwhile, the city's waste disposal systems hadn't evolved in two hundred years. As you might imagine, running a veritable farm out of your studio apartment could produce a lot of waste. People had cesspools in their basements, where they disposed of their feces and urine—human and animal. According to Steven Johnson, the author of *The Ghost Map: The Story of London's Most Terrifying Epidemic—and How It Changed Science, Cities, and the Modern World*, "They would just kind of throw the buckets down there and hope that it would somehow go away and of course it would never really go away."[6] Ugh, of course it did not. The amount of feces abounding in London did lend itself to an economy, though. "Pure Finders" roamed the street collecting dog poop, which they sold to tanners, who would smear it on leather skins to remove lime from them. As happy as I am that the Pure Finders managed to make money, I don't think anyone wants to live in a city with such an abundant shit supply.

Although diseases don't stem from "bad smells," some are carried by insects and other pests that are drawn to excrement and other creators of bad odors. So cleaning up your cesspools and removing fecal matter from the street are good ideas in general. *Unless* your solution is to dump the waste into the River Thames.

Everyone drank from the Thames, and it was now filled with decades' worth of fecal matter and urine from people's basements. In 1850 Charles Dickens described the river, lamenting that it was "the black contents of common sewers and the refuse of gut, glue, soap and other nauseous manufactures, to say nothing of animal and vegetable offal of which the river is the sole receptacle."[7] In 1853 an article in the *Builder* declared: "The flood . . . is now, below London Bridge, bad as poetical descriptions of the Stygian Lake, while the London Dock is black as Acheron . . . where are ye, ye civil engineers? Ye can remove mountains, bridge seas and fill rivers . . . can ye not purify the Thames, and so render your own city habitable?"[8] Drinking from such a river is a truly terrible plan if you do not wish to die.

Especially if you're dealing with a cholera outbreak. In fact, cholera was the main problem that the Nuisances Act was hoping to address. However, cholera isn't spread through the smells in the air, as officials thought. It is spread through ingesting other people's infected defecated matter. If you are thinking, *I'm not into that. Even the idea of that is disgusting to me on a primal level,* you are an evolved human being. The thought is so repulsive to most people that the whole horror movie trilogy *The Human Centipede* (2009–15) is based on the premise "What if people had to eat other people's shit? That'd be a real bummer!" (Sorry I spoiled the movies, but you probably saw the best bits in the Academy Award recaps anyway.)

While almost no one would contract it on purpose, cholera is very easy to acquire unintentionally if you are drinking water contaminated with fecal matter. Enough cholera bacteria to kill a person wouldn't even cloud the water you were drinking. Once you have drunk it *without even knowing it,* the cholera bacterium settles in the small intestine. There, it begins reproducing and forms a toxin called CTX, which covers the walls of the small intestines. Now, the main purpose of the small intestine is to keep you hydrated; it absorbs water and then sends it on to other areas of the body. However, when its walls are coated with cholera bacteria, it instead begins expelling water. The result is a white-flaked, watery diarrhea that is referred to as "rice stool." Cool fact: the "rice" flakes are actually cells from the small intestine. People would expel so much water that they could lose 30 percent of their body weight. Someone would drop from a healthy 120 pounds to a deadly 85 pounds within days. Without water, first nonessential organs begin to shut down, and then the essential organs like the heart and kidneys fail. The brain, perhaps especially tragically, was often the last organ to succumb, so people would remain conscious of their suffering until the end. The British newspaper the *Times* claimed that it gave people in the throes of death the appearance of "a spirit looking out in terror from a corpse."[9] Then the deceased's cholera-contaminated rice stool would be dumped into the river or nearby water supply (or cesspool in the cases where people still insisted on having them, despite the Nuisances Act), and the process would be repeated.

If the above paragraph was too long: People shat themselves to death. It was, and still is in countries where clean water is not readily available, a *horrible* way to die.

But into this literally shitty quagmire stepped a hero. He was a physician named John Snow, and, like the *Game of Thrones* character Jon Snow, he was a real square. He was self-righteous in all his habits. He was a fervent teetotaler. Which is fine! The most accomplished people I know never drink and are always getting up early to run marathons. But Snow wrote very long, dry speeches on how you—you fool—should not drink alcohol. One that he wrote at the wise old age of twenty-three explains: "I feel it my duty to endeavour to convince you of the physical evils sustained to your health by using intoxicating liquors even in the greatest moderation; and I leave to my colleagues the task of painting drunkenness in all its hideousness, of describing the manifold miseries and crimes it produces, and of proving to you that total abstinence is the only remedy for those evils."[10] I am positive he would give that speech every time you had a glass of wine at dinner. He also claimed that people drank because of a level of curiosity "unpossessed of which we should remain as stationary as brutes; and which, if allowed to lie dormant, would cause us to remain for generations with as little improvement as the Chinese."[11] I thought he was going to say "as little improvement as animals," but I was wrong! The fact that he hated the

Chinese was not all that unusual by nineteenth-century British standards, but it doesn't make me like him *more*. In any event, his fervent antialcoholism is ironic given that this was perhaps the only period in history when from a health standpoint you would have been better off consuming alcohol than water.

I am not exaggerating or joking when I make that statement. In one instance, during the cholera epidemic of 1854 all eighty workers at a London brewery notably managed to avoid catching the disease. To be fair, the brewery had its own well, but the proprietor noted that most of the men just drank the liquor they produced.[12]

Snow was also a vegan, though it "puzzled the housewives, shocked the cooks and astonished the children."[13] Again, being a vegan is cool—good for him—but I will bet you every penny I have that he never shut up about it. He was known to have a poor bedside manner and almost no social life. He wrote so many critical articles that at one point the editor of the *Lancet* journal wrote, "Mr. Snow might better employ himself in producing something, than in criticizing the production of others."[14] His acquaintance and later biographer Dr. Benjamin Ward Richardson noted: "He took no wine nor strong drink; he lived on anchorite's fare, clothed plainly, kept no company, and found every amusement in his science books, his experiments and simple exercise."[15]

Sounds super fun.

Okay. He may not be the hero we wanted, but he is the one we got. Let us fete him with a stick of celery and some seltzer.

There were many times when being antisocial and extremely critical didn't work in Snow's favor. Having him as a guest for dinner sounds like a nightmare. (Playing "What three historical figures would you most *hate* to have dinner with?" is an amusing variation on the "Which people living or dead would you like to dine with?" game.) However, Snow's cantankerous personality proved useful when going against everyone else, who had agreed upon a theory that was literally killing them. John Snow's refusal to go merrily along with the rest of his profession's assertion that cholera was spread either by the miasma theory or from person-to-person contagion proved very valuable.

Snow had treated an outbreak of cholera in 1832, so he was well aware of its devastating effects.[16] However, it was in 1848, during an outbreak that killed fifty thousand people in England and Wales, that Snow traced the first case in London to a sick sailor traveling from Hamburg. The sailor died in a room at a boardinghouse in London. That room was then occupied by another man, who also caught cholera and died. Now, I know what you are thinking, you nineteenth-century miasmist: *This was truly a remarkable coincidence! Both Hamburg and London must smell terrible right now. How unfortunate.* Everyone in the medical profession would have agreed with you. However, it seemed more likely to Snow that cholera had been transmitted in some way by the sailor from Hamburg, especially since he was coming from a city where the disease was killing people. Okay, that might indicate it could be passed from person to person. But the sailor was already dead (and gone) by the time the second inhabitant moved into the room. The doctor who had visited both these men never contracted cholera. Snow noticed that often doctors from different neighborhoods could visit with cholera patients but never get the disease themselves. Meanwhile, sometimes an entire neighborhood would be struck down.

Snow determined that people were somehow *ingesting* the disease and were being made sick by "morbid matter," although he wasn't precisely sure how.

By 1849 he was convinced cholera was spread by water. He had studied a group of twelve people who lived in a row of cottages and who had all contracted the disease. The people in the next row of cottages—who were surely exposed to the same smells in the air, and with whom the residents of the first cottages mingled—remained perfectly healthy. He found that the well for the first row of cottages was cracked; its water supply was being contaminated by a nearby sewer. The people in the second row of cottages pulled their water from a different well. Snow also noted that, while the East End of London smelled terrible, it didn't have nearly the same number of cholera cases as South London, where people received much of their water from a particularly contaminated area of the Thames.[17]

Our hero published a paper on these findings, which you and I would probably find wholly convincing as we already know that Snow was correct. However, people of that time did not believe his theory at all. According to the *London Medical Gazette*: "Other causes, irrespective of the water, may have been in operation especially as the persons were living in close proximity . . . The facts here mentioned raise only a probability, and furnish no proof whatsoever of the author's views."[18] Proof, according to the journal, would depend on one source of water that, when conveyed to a community "where cholera had been hitherto unknown, produced the disease in all who used it, while those who did not use it escaped."[19]

So John Snow waited for an outbreak where such a case might be found. He practiced anesthesiology in the meantime, and he was great at it—he was present at the birth of two of Queen Victoria's children. He was probably so proficient because *he was a total snooze.* (Why am I so mean to this good man who just wanted to save lives?)

Faulty assumptions about the nature of cholera might have gone on forever if, on August 28, 1854, an infant known as Baby Lewis (her real name was Frances) had not contracted the disease. It's not known how the baby got cholera. However, it is known that her family lived at 40 Broad Street, which had a cesspool in front that, unfortunately for everyone in London, bordered on the most popular water pump in Soho—the Broad Street pump. This pump was famous for the high quality of its water; it had such a good reputation that even people who didn't live nearby would use it for their water supply. So it's unfortunate that once her baby contracted cholera, Mrs. Lewis tossed Frances's filthy excrement into that cesspool, where it began contaminating the pump's water supply.

Though the water from the pump was barely discolored, the cholera bacterium began its deadly work. Seventy-four people in the neighborhood died by September 3. Hundreds more were on the verge of death. Within a week, 10 percent of the neighborhood was dead,[20] including Frances's father. Although cholera often killed devastating numbers of people in a memorably agonizing way, it didn't usually work so quickly. Typically, it took months to kill the hundreds of people who, in this instance, died within days.

Snow lived only a few blocks away from the neighborhood. While other residents of Soho fled to stay with friends in different areas of town, he eagerly began his investigation. "As soon as I became acquainted with the situation and extent of this irruption of cholera," he wrote, "I suspected some contamination of the water of the much-frequented street-pump in Broad Street."[21]

But how to go about proving his theory? Snow began going through the neighborhood and questioning the inhabitants about the habits of everyone who had acquired cholera. He constructed a map charting the outbreak, and in doing so noticed that the closer people were to the Broad Street pump, the more likely they were to be sick or dead. Those who did not get cholera had their own wells or, for whatever reason, chose not to use the Broad Street pump.

Not all of the cases were obvious, of course. A few people didn't recall drinking water from the pump; however, they *had* consumed sherbet, which was sold on the street and made from water from the pump. Another woman lived in Hampstead, absolutely nowhere near the Broad Street pump, and yet she had still contracted cholera. So had her niece who was staying with her. This would seem to contradict Snow's theory, if not for the fact that the woman had formerly lived in Soho and believed the

water from the Broad Street pump was *the best*. That is a charming bit of sentimental attachment to your former neighborhood.
Her son explained to Snow that she loved the water so much that
her children periodically bottled it and sent it to her in care
packages. That lady's inadvertently murderous family sounds so
sweet and caring, and I feel very sad for them.

But I'm guessing Snow was at least pleased on an intellectual
level. Finally, here was the proof that the *London Medical Gazette*
had claimed was necessary to prove that cholera was carried by
water! In this case the water had quite literally been moved to a
community "where cholera had been hitherto unknown, [and]
produced the disease in all who used it." The Hampstead cases
could not simply be explained by the sickly smelling air around
the Broad Street pump.

On September 7, Snow shared his findings with town officials and implored them to remove the handle from the Broad
Street pump. He explained the high rate of disease around
the pump and how even people far removed from the pump
who had drunk from the same water supply became sick. On
September 8, the handle to the Broad Street pump was removed.
Today, this breakthrough is the stuff of legend, so much so that
when officials at the Centers for Disease Control and Prevention
are looking for a solution to a medical mystery, they are known
to joke, "Where's the handle to the Broad Street pump?"[22]

No sooner did the cases of cholera decline than people began
to look for alternate reasons for the abatement. On September 15
the *Times* reported that around Soho there was

> a continual presence of [the strong smelling disinfect] lime
> in the roadways. The puddles are white and milky with it, the
> stones are smeared with it; great splashes of it lie about in
> the gutters, and the air is redolent with its strong and not
> very agreeable odor. The parish authorities have very wisely
> determined to wash all the streets of the tainted district with

this powerful disinfectant; accordingly the purification takes place regularly every evening.[23]

That had . . . nothing to do with why cholera was subsiding, although the fact that the streets were being made to smell of cleaning chemicals rather than more disagreeable odors would certainly satisfy those who believed in the miasma theory.

The *Globe*, meanwhile, attributed the decline as "owing to the favourable change in the weather, the pestilence which has raged with such frightful severity in this district has abated, and it may be hoped that the inhabitants have seen the worst of the visitation."[24] No. Wrong again. But it was so much easier for people to think that bad odors—which they could smell and experience themselves—caused disease than to believe that it was due to something invisible in the water.

In March 1855 Snow was called upon for testimony regarding an amendment to the Nuisances Act, which hoped to regulate industries like gas workers and bone boilers. Those industries emitted disgusting fumes into the air. So Snow was put in what must have been a peculiar position of defending the rights of industry to render bones, which, while gross, was not actually causing cholera. His testimony gave him the opportunity to strike down the miasma theory:

> I have paid a great deal of attention to epidemic diseases, more particularly to cholera, and in fact to the public health in general; and I have arrived at the conclusion with regard to what are called offensive trades, that many of them really do not assist in the propagation of epidemic diseases, and that in fact they are not injurious to the public health. I consider that if they were injurious to the public health they would be extremely so to the workmen engaged in those trades, and as far as I have been able to learn, that is not the case; and from the law of the diffusion of gases, it follows, that if

they are not injurious to those actually upon the spot, where the trades are carried on, it is impossible they should be to persons further removed from the spot.[25]

One interesting and weirdly specific aspect of the discussion was when Snow was asked why, if smells can't make you sick, do people vomit if they smell something extremely bad? Specifically, the chairman Benjamin Hall questioned, "I understand you to say that such effluvia, when highly concentrated, may produce vomiting, but that they are not injurious to health. How do you reconcile those two propositions?"

If you have the same question, today it's thought that noxious smells act on a receptor in the nose that warns your body of impending danger.[26] A caveman in an area rife with bad smells is probably in an area where there are predators. The physical response tells his body to get out. Snow said only that he thought "it might be a kind of sympathy. Persons are often much influenced by the imagination," but the important aspect was that smells do not make people permanently sick: "If the vomiting were repeatedly produced, it would certainly be injurious to health. If a person was constantly exposed to decomposing matter, so concentrated as to disturb the digestive organs, it must be admitted that that would be injurious to health; but I am not aware that, in following any useful trade or manufacture, the effects ever experienced."[27]

Basically, if something smells so bad it makes you vomit uncontrollably, you should probably leave the room. The fact that the people at this hearing harped on an irrelevant question reminds me of the days after 9/11 when, as I think Jon Stewart mentioned at the time, newscasters began postulating increasingly outlandish scenarios, like "What would happen if a terrorist had a smart bomb shaped exactly like a donut and the president ate it?" Well, it would be bad, but it was also not going to happen. Similarly, no one was going to remain in a room where bad smells made them vomit until they died. "Why do smells make people vomit then, huh, huh?" feels like the last desperate attempts of officials to hold on to their "known" world.

They were holding on hard. Some were still unmoved and furious. Medical journals like the *Lancet* were especially withering. The editor wrote of Snow:

> Why is it, then, that Dr. Snow is so singular in his opinion? Has he any facts to show in proof? No! . . . But Dr. Snow claims to have discovered that the law of propagation of cholera is the drinking of the sewage-water. His theory, of course, displaces all other theories. Other theories [that] attribute great efficacy in the spread of cholera to bad drainage and vegetable decomposition are innocuous! If this logic does not satisfy reason, it satisfies a theory; and we all know that theory is often more despotic than reason. The fact is, that the well whence Dr. Snow draws all sanitary truth is the main sewer. His specus, or den, is a drain. In riding his hobby very hard, he has fallen down through a gully-hole and has never since been able to get out again.[28]

First of all, it's surprising to see a medical journal declaring "He lives in a metaphorical sewer!" of a fellow doctor. I guess the medical profession was filled with more vim and vigor and public hatred then. Beyond that, Snow had many facts to show proof. He made a map! He did study after study! He spent his life doing absolutely nothing except accumulating facts to prove his theory on the cause of cholera, dosing people with chloroform, and eating uncooked vegetables. His life was defined by his relentless dedication to combatting cholera. Richardson wrote, "No one but those who knew him intimately can conceive how he labored, at what cost, and at what risk. Wherever cholera was visitant, there was he in the midst."[29]

Saying Snow did not have his facts in order was groundless. Although I would never have dinner with the man, I will defend to the death the statement that Snow's investigative research was impeccable.

But his opponents persisted. The public health activist Edwin Chadwick and the president of the Board of Health Benjamin Hall denounced Snow's reasoning. Snow's rebuttal in a letter to Hall declared: "Although there is sufficient direct evidence to prove that cholera is neither caused nor increased by offensive trades, that circumstance is very much confirmed by the facts which I have been able to collect in illustration of the mode of propagation of cholera; for it is not reasonable to seek for additional causes of any phenomenon, when a real and adequate cause is known."[30] He does not know why you keep trying to find other causes for a disease when he has *told you the cause.*

Another detractor skeptical of Snow's theory was Reverend Henry Whitehead. The twenty-nine-year-old curate of St. Luke's Church in the Soho neighborhood was convinced of the miasma theory. He claimed "an extensive inquiry would reveal the falsity of the Snow hypothesis regarding the Broad Street pump."[31]

If you have ever read the comments under a medical article online (oh, God, do not, please do not; you will get so angry your head will explode, and you need your brain), you will know that many people think that in boldly making a claim—any claim— their point is proven, and that they can sit back smugly secure in the fact that it has been established that they are smarter than the author-doctor-scientist.

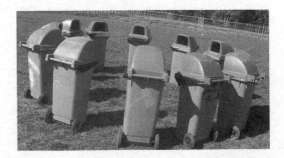

Cool group photo of those commenters

But Reverend Whitehead was not an Internet commenter. He was a man of God who had ethics as well as bold convictions. He meticulously interviewed everyone in the Soho neighborhood, sometimes reviewing their information four or five times. He completed an even more elaborate map than Snow's, which took into account everyone who had left the neighborhood and been hospitalized elsewhere, and all the people who had visited the area and then became sick. "Slowly and I may add reluctantly," he concluded, "that the use of water [from the Broad Street pump] was connected with the continuation of the outburst."[32] He became such a firm convert to Snow's theory that until his death Whitehead kept over his desk a portrait of Snow, which, he noted, "ever serves to remind me that in any profession the highest order of work is achieved not by fussy demand for 'something to be done,' but by patient study of the eternal laws."[33] Whitehead published his findings in June 1855 in the article "Special Investigation of Broad Street." Only then did the medical committee of the General Board of Health decide that the outbreak of cholera "lasting for the few early days in September was in some manner attributable to the use of the impure water of the well in Broad Street."[34] The committee members were nearly evenly split on that decision.

Skepticism persisted for years. As late as 1859 the *Lancet* claimed that there was absolutely no doubt that noxious smells were "a most efficient and malignant influence in the causation and aggravation of disease."[35] However, in 1866, during the next outbreak of cholera, officials told citizens that they should begin boiling their water. You know, just in case John Snow was right.

There was never another cholera outbreak in London.

Ever.

The local government board declared in 1866 that "the remarkable and shrewd observations of Dr. Snow, demonstrat[ed] incontrovertibly the connexion of cholera with a consumption of specifically polluted water."[36]

John Snow, sadly, never witnessed the public validation of his theory. He died in 1858 of a reported stroke. Possibly! There is a rumor that the cause of death was not a stroke and instead an overdose as he was allegedly always dosing himself with anesthesia, which would be a genuinely surprising habit for such a fervent teetotaler.

In that same year a heat wave caused the river—and the city surrounding it—to reek so badly that the phenomenon was referred to as "the Great Stink." That summer, it was also found that the rate of death from diseases like cholera had not spiked, even with the many terrible smells in the air. Snow would have been delighted; I am sincerely sad he did not live to see the miasma theory waft away.

Snow's obituary in the *Lancet* did not mention his cholera findings. It only read: "This well-known physician died at noon on the 16th instant, at his house in Sackville-street, from an attack of apoplexy. His researches on chloroform and other anaesthetics were appreciated by the profession."[37] But by 1866 the journal declared: "The researches of Dr. Snow are among the most fruitful in modern medicine. He traced the history of cholera. We owe to him chiefly the severe induction by which the influence of the poisoning of water-supplies was proved. No greater service could be rendered to humanity than this; it has enabled us to meet and combat the disease, where alone it is to be vanquished, in its sources or channels of propagation . . . Dr. Snow was a great public benefactor, and the benefits which he conferred must be fresh in the minds of all."[38] That's very nice. However, this praise ran beside an article regarding the 1866 outbreak in which *some dude* (okay, Mr. Orton, a medical officer) claimed he had "facts which induce him to believe that the local nuisances have had their part quite as well as the water in production of cholera."[39]

There are always going to be some people who believe that the sun is revolving around a flat earth.

Today, John Snow is a medical legend. As for him being boring company, well, Dr. Richardson, Snow's biographer, hammers home my shallowness in his preface to Snow's *On Chloroform and Other Anaesthetics: Their Action and Administration* (1858). Richardson remarks that a biography of Snow would "be scanty in its details; it is of but little count that the life of him who is about to be shadowed forth is destitute of incident fitted for the taste of wonder-loving, passion-courting, romance-devouring readers. Biographies for these are common. Good men are scarce."[40]

Okay, Dr. Richardson. I get it. Still, you may be delighted to know that in Snow's memory, there is now an institution named after him by the site of the Broad Street pump in London. *It is a pub.* The owner must either have known nothing about Snow's personal character or had a really keen, beautiful sense of humor.

If you genuinely want to celebrate John Snow and you are in London, go in and raise a glass to him. It should be a glass full of clean, cool, feces-free water. It's what Snow would have wanted.

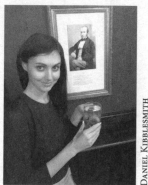

DANIEL KIBBLESMITH

Cheers, guys.

Leprosy

*The biggest disease today is not
leprosy or tuberculosis, but rather the
feeling of being unwanted, uncared
for, and deserted by everybody.*

—Mother Teresa

The best-case scenario when it comes to the outbreak of a
disease is that the community will rally around the afflicted. It
will tend to them gently; it will raise funds; it will do whatever
is necessary to allow the people stricken with the disease to live
with dignity while science searches for a cure. When the community as a whole swings into action, plagues can be overcome
relatively swiftly.

That almost never happens.

But, fortunately, it doesn't always take an entire community.
Every so often there is an outsider who is willing to take on the
caregiving of the diseased. Maybe you're thinking, *Well, I would
do that, but I am not a doctor.* But you don't have to be a doctor!
Groups of people doing walks to benefit disease research in
brightly colored T-shirts come to mind, as do elegantly attired

people hosting events to raise funds. And, though he wasn't as impressively attired, so does that shining nineteenth-century example of compassion and humanity—Father Damien of Molokai.

Guided by his faith, Father Damien chose to live among the lepers on the island of Molokai as their priest, assisting them practically and spiritually and, while doing so, contracted leprosy himself. In 2009 he was canonized by Pope Benedict XVI, who claimed: "Father Damien made the choice to go on the island of Molokai in the service of lepers who were there, abandoned by all. So he exposed himself to the disease of which they suffered. With them he felt at home. The servant of the Word became a suffering servant, leper with the lepers, during the last four years of his life."[1] Damien's sainthood prompted President Barack Obama to remark: "In our own time as millions around the world suffer from disease, especially the pandemic of HIV/AIDS, we should draw on the example of Father Damien's resolve in answering the urgent call to heal and care for the sick."[2] That comment is especially applicable today as Damien is the unofficial patron saint of those suffering from HIV/AIDS; the sole Catholic memorial chapel to the victims of HIV and AIDS is dedicated to him.[3]

Leprosy, the disease Father Damien gave his life to fighting, is terrifying in an epic way. People have been very afraid of it from the beginning of recorded history. It is mentioned in the Bible, where it is often associated with sin. Leviticus 13:45–46 says: "And the leper in whom the plague [is], his clothes shall be rent, and his head bare, and he shall put a covering upon his upper lip, and shall cry, Unclean, unclean. All the days wherein the plague [shall be] in him he shall be defiled; he [is] unclean: he shall dwell alone; without the camp [shall] his habitation [be]."[4]

Sunday school teachings notwithstanding, this is not true. Leprosy has nothing to do with whether someone has a shiny, clean soul or body. *No* diseases have anything to do with anyone's soul. Leprosy is a bacterial disease, caused by *Mycobacterium leprae.* The Norwegian doctor Gerhard Hansen identified the bacterial cause in 1873, and the disease today is often called Hansen's disease. However, he is not going to be a hero in this story, and I refuse to refer to leprosy by that term because in the course of his research he *infected a woman with full-blown leprosy without her knowledge.*[5] He claimed he didn't tell her what he was going to do because he couldn't "presuppose that the patient would regard the experiment from the same point of view as I myself did."[6]

No, perhaps not, Gerhard.

The *Mycobacterium leprae* can pass into a body through an open cut or through mucous membranes in the nose. That seems like an easy way to become infected, but the good news is that most individuals aren't especially susceptible to the disease. To contract it, people have to be in constant, close contact with lepers.

Leprosy manifests in two ways. The first is *tuberculoid leprosy,* where rough, scaly lesions develop over the skin. That's because the disease sets off a cellular reaction in which immune cells rush to isolate the bacteria. The reaction spreads to the nerves in the affected areas and stops nerve signals from being transmitted, so sufferers lose sensation at that site. Sometimes this kind of leprosy resolves, though in other cases it progresses and turns into *lepromatous leprosy.* In those cases, the bacteria spread all over the body, causing open sores on the face and body. In some cases, the disease also leads to blindness.

The most notable feature of leprosy—and in many cases the first symptom of the disease—is the loss of the sense of touch. That doesn't sound terrible until you realize that if you are accidentally walking over broken glass, it is good to know that. It's also good to know if you burned yourself or chopped off your finger while cooking or otherwise injured yourself in a way that should be tended to. And the injuries don't have to be that extreme to cause problems! With no feeling in your limbs, you could just not notice an everyday blister from too-tight shoes and continue walking around in those shoes until the sore becomes infected. It's because of the resulting infections from these injuries that lepers came to be associated with missing fingers, hands, or feet—the bacterium itself doesn't actually cause them to fall off. However, it does cause muscles to weaken in a way that results in deformities. For instance, lepers are often thought to have hands that look like claws. That's because the muscles in their hands are no longer strong enough to extend their fingers.

Today, like many historical plagues, leprosy can be treated with antibiotics, which are provided for free by the World Health Organization. It is yet another disease that, if you have enough resources at your disposal to buy and read this book, you are never going to need to worry about. But it understandably terrified people of the past. Because the symptoms of the disease were so obvious, the people who had it were regarded as outcasts. In fact, some people thought the best way to fight the disease was to make sure no one had contact with any lepers at all.

In 1865 the Hawaiian government enacted "An Act to Prevent the Spread of Leprosy." It claimed that a portion of land—which would end up being on the island of Molokai—would be set aside for leprous individuals. This is where it got scary:

> The Board of Health or its agents are authorized and empowered to cause to be confined, in some place or places for that purpose provided, all leprous patients who shall be deemed capable of spreading the disease of leprosy . . . it shall be the duty of the Marshal of the Hawaiian Islands and his deputies, and of the police officers, to assist in securing the conveyance of any person so arrested to such place, as the Board of Health, or its agents may direct, in order that such person

may be subjected to medical inspection, and thereafter to assist in removing such person to place of treatment or isolation, if so required, by the agents of the Board of Health.[7]

In short, if you were suspected of being a leper, the government was going to hunt you down and forcibly move you off to quarantine.

If this policy does not strike you as desirable or in any way okay, you are not alone. There is even a Jack London story, called "Koolau the Leper," in which the protagonist is a leper who would rather fight and die than go to Molokai. The story begins with him saying: "Because we are sick they take away our liberty. We have obeyed the law. We have done no wrong. And yet they would put us in prison. Molokai is a prison."[8]

I would have gone with *hellhole* rather than *prison*, but however you phrase it, conditions on Molokai were dire. The government hoped that the lepers would take care of themselves, farming the land and living off their own resources, seemingly forgetting how hard that is to do if people do not have all of their extremities intact. Moreover, the lepers were depressed about being suddenly cast out of society. If you isolate people from their families and friends when they have a serious disease, physical disabilities, and very little hope, they understandably may not behave really well.

I would probably have responded to that situation by becoming a severe alcoholic and having a lot of sex to try to distract myself from the daily misery of my condition and surroundings. Maybe you would have done better, but many seemed to share my feelings. In 1913 the missionary Joseph Dutton wrote in the *Catholic Encyclopedia*, volume 10: "Matters went on pretty well at first, but after some time an ugly spirit developed at Molokai. Drunken and lewd conduct prevailed. The easy-going, good-natured people seemed wholly changed."[9]

Arriving at the colony was like being plunged into some sort of heartbreaking dystopia. In *Leper Priest of Molokai: The Father Damien Story*, Richard Stewart writes of the medical facilities: "Conspicuously absent in the so-called hospital were doctors, nurses and a supply of medicines with which to treat the more common diseases that plagued the lepers and precipitated their demise . . . water for cleaning the open sores and bathing was in disturbingly short supply."[10] Some doctors would not touch their patients and lifted their bandages with a cane. Others just left medicine where the lepers could access it and refused to have any contact with them at all.[11]

If you treat people like monsters, they behave that way. Dutton wasn't exaggerating. The island was filled with crime, drunkenness, and abuses of every kind. Damien later reported that "many an unfortunate woman had to become a prostitute in order to obtain friends who would take care of her." This wasn't just the fate of grown women; child prostitutes abounded on the island.[12] And, as Damien went on to say, "once the disease prostrated them, such women and children were cast out."[13] So there were outcasts even among the lepers. If you visited Molokai, you would hear the phrase "A 'ole kanawai ma keia wahi" with some regularity. It means, "In this place there is no law."[14] There was—comically—a jail, but it stood empty because no one was able to enforce rules.[15]

I think a universal human fear is that we will die alone. To die, even in the absolute best possible situation, is to set off on a very big journey, and everyone deserves kind people around to see them off. I cannot imagine a more lonely place to die than Molokai prior to Damien's arrival. Molokai needed a priest.

Damien wasn't always godly; he wasn't even always Damien. He was born Jozef (Jef) de Veuster in Tremelo, Belgium, in 1840. He was a nice kid. His family was religious, and his mother enjoyed telling the stories of the lives of saints, but family piety didn't stop mischievous Damien from hitching joyrides on the back of horse-drawn wagons[16] or skating around on thin ice during the winter, much to his family's concern.[17] He was kind to animals and the less fortunate; he once stole a ham from his mother's kitchen and gave it to a beggar, which, again, didn't really thrill his family.[18] He helped his neighbor nurse her sick cow back to health.[19] I want to imagine his family was okay with that and maybe received some free milk.

In 1858, when he was age nineteen, he sought to begin his religious training. At his admission interview he said he hoped to work as a missionary in North America among the Native Americans. That is a cool answer. I think it is good to remember that cowboys were fashionably hip at the time, and I'm glad Damien picked the underdog in the traditional cowboy-Indian fight. However, I suspect he was not supposed to say "I'd like to travel and experience new cultures" as his reason for wanting to be a priest (that is only a good response on your college-year-abroad application). He was initially rejected by the Congregation of the Sacred Hearts of Jesus and Mary, in Louvain, where his older brother Auguste (Father Pamphile) was studying to become a priest. Jef was considered unsuitable because of his "rudeness in manner and appearance and ignorance of Latin and any other language."[20]

You know how people periodically bring up the fact that Einstein failed mathematics, to reassure parents that even though their child is receiving Ds and Fs in every math class, he or she still has the potential to figure out the theory of relativity? Three points:

1. That story about Einstein is probably a lie; he was generally a superb student.
2. As someone whose mother heard that story a lot, I can assure you that the only math an average human needs is how to calculate a 20 percent tip on a check, and you're allowed to use your iPhone calculator; no one will laugh at you for doing so.

3. I still hope Father Damien's story will be similarly comforting to anyone who wants to be a missionary but is turned down by the religious school of his choosing.

After some begging and pleading on his brother's part, Jef was eventually admitted to the congregation as a choir brother. Choir brothers could possibly, *maybe,* become priests. However, it was more likely that they would simply remain at the monastery helping with daily tasks and studying the Bible in their spare time, which sounds great! Really quiet and low-key and peaceful and nonthreatening. I bet there was a lot of gardening involved and also some cooking, reading, and singing—just an ideal retirement, honestly. I guess not everyone felt that way. The positions were considered a place in the religious order for—sorry, choir brothers—nice guys who didn't seem quite smart or charismatic enough to be out among the people preaching the word of God.[21] Jef entered the order and adopted the name Brother Damien, after the third-century physician Damian, who refused to accept payment for his services.[22]

Surprisingly to the order if not to you, modern reader, Damien exceeded everyone's expectations. His brother taught him Latin, and I have a personal theory that Damien was one of those sleepless elites who only needed four hours of rest a night. He would pray before the altar beginning at two or three in the morning and didn't go back to bed afterward. Within a year, he had the skill of a fifth-year Latin student and could translate on sight. The only fault the monks seemed to find with him was that he laughed too much. In spite of Damien being so cool and hilarious, it was decided by the seminary superior that he should begin training for the priesthood after all.[23]

By 1863 Damien wasn't yet a priest, but his brother had recently been made one. Pamphile's first assignment was to work as a missionary in Hawaii. However, shortly before Pamphile was to depart, he became sick with typhus. He recovered but was too ill to go on a long sea voyage. Brother Damien asked to take his place, saying that he could finish up his studies en route. When his request was granted, he supposedly burst into his brother's room shouting, "Yes! Yes! I am to go instead of you! I am to go instead of you!"[24]

So many biographers respond to this event by claiming, "Oh, how happy this must have made Pamphile." I don't know what those biographers' childhoods were like, but this is *exactly* like running into your sibling's room with a Disneyland ticket and screaming, "Guess where I'm going!" when your sibling is sick in bed with chicken pox. Damien was such a jackass here. I still like him a lot, and if you've ever been similarly insufferable, it's nice to know that this behavior won't rule you out for sainthood.

Things worked out fine for Pamphile, by the way. He served as instructor to novices—or new arrivals—to the congregation. It was a high-ranking position that, Damien wrote in a letter, meant he was "raised in dignity," although Damien had hoped his brother might join him as a missionary.

Damien was assigned to a ministry in Kohala, where, he claimed, "visiting the sick is one of my chief duties each day."[25] Preaching in Hawaii meant that he soon heard stories about the "Kalaupapa prison,"[26] as the Kalaupapa peninsula on the Island of Molokai, which housed the leper colony, was sometimes called. The lepers there had been writing to the church begging for a priest for some time. The bishop Maigret assembled a group to discuss the problem, though he held out little hope that anyone would volunteer for the dangerous and unappealing assignment. However, Damien and three other priests thought that they could serve on the island in rotation, each spending around three months there each year. Even once Damien departed, in 1873, the bishop was still concerned, famously writing that Damien could stay "as long as [his] devotion dictates."[27] He likely meant to give Damien an easy out; instead, Damien seemed to take it as the permission he needed to remain at Molokai for the next sixteen years.

Before Damien's departure, the bishop explained the protocol of dealing with the lepers. According to Stewart: "There was to be no physical contact with a leper . . . his priests would never eat food prepared by a leper, nor would a priest ever sleep in a leper's house."[28] The bishop was especially clear that Damien must "never touch or allow [him]self to be touched by a leper."[29] Moreover, if any of the afflicted offered him a smoking pipe, he must refuse it, and he should not sit with them for any communal meals or even use a saddle that a leper had previously used.[30] He was more or less there to read them their last rites, and that was *it*.

Damien disobeyed the bishop's instructions the minute he landed on the peninsula. He was greeted by a religious leper who offered him fruit, which he gratefully accepted. And presumably ate.[31]

Shortly thereafter he began visiting each of the lepers' homes. At one he found a young girl whose wounds were so untended that worms covered the side of her body.[32] Damien started changing the lepers' bandages by hand.[33] I suspect as soon as Damien saw that girl, he knew that he couldn't make life bearable for the people of Molokai if he wasn't willing to risk dying. He might have known that as soon as he set foot on the island, really. I would like to think that you and I would come to the same conclusion, but I am 100 percent certain I would not do the same. My devotion to my fellow man does not extend to treating wounds crawling with worms. Maybe yours does! If you are a missionary reading this book, I think you are getting a fast-pass to heaven, and I am really sorry about all the swear words I have used.

Damien wrote a lot about his affection and respect for the lepers. However, he did also write, "Sometimes, confessing the sick, whose sores are full of worms like cadavers in the grave, I have to hold my nose."[34] Damien strikes me as so superhuman in his goodness that it's relieving to stumble across an incident that reminds us that he was still a regular person sensitive to smell and worms. Supposedly, whenever he was lonely or frightened on the island, he would spur himself on by repeating to himself, "Come on, Jef, my boy, this is your life's work!"

Church services began shortly after Damien's arrival at the Chapel of St. Philomena. When Damien arrived the chapel was squalid, and he spent hours cleaning it out.[35] The pandanus tree next to the church served as the chapel's first rectory; a rock was his dinner table.[36] As he made contact with more lepers, Damien obtained their help in improving the church, encouraging them to build alongside him. Soon it became a center not just of religion but for all manner of activities. The community was organized into a congregation. The area around the church served as a gravesite, where Damien conducted funerals, a welcome and compassionate improvement on how the lepers' bodies had often been abandoned without ceremony before.[37] A church choir was formed, despite the fact that, owing to the weakened vocal cords of many sufferers, the songs didn't always come out as intended. The church organist had lost his left hand but attached a piece of wood to the stump in order to play all the organ's notes. Occasionally two people would play the organ, as between them they had enough fingers to hit every key.[38]

These stories might seem dark to us, but to lepers who had felt forsaken for so long, belonging to a community again must have been wonderful. It's completely fair to say that the lepers' band would never have been featured on the *Late Show*, but that wasn't really the point. The lepers knew that their lives would never go back to "normal." What the lepers surely wanted was to be able to participate in some way in the activities they had enjoyed before contracting their disease and, in doing so, to perhaps have a few minutes when they felt like their old, normal selves again. Maybe that's what everyone suffering from a disease wants. So when Damien noted at a foot race that one man failed to "toe the mark" because he had no toes, it was a cause for laughter, not despair. The fact that the flutes Damien distributed often had to be played with an inadequate number of fingers didn't mean that people didn't enjoy playing them.[39]

When he wasn't making bad jokes at foot races, Damien labored to eradicate some of the practical terrors that had afflicted the island. Tackling the problem of inadequate water, he worked with the healthiest lepers to create a dam that collected the rainwater streaming down the side of a cliff. That water was used for drinking and medical purposes, but also to irrigate crops like taro, sweet potatoes, and sugarcane, which Damien and the more able-bodied lepers planted.[40]

There were risks. An issue of the *Journal of the American Medical Association* explained: "The manual labor of the roughest kind which he did for the lepers, to make them more comfortable, could not fail to produce frequently cuts, punctures and abrasions, by which the danger of inoculation was greatly increased."[41] But Damien didn't seem much concerned. He was thrilled that by 1886, 90 percent of the residents of the peninsula had begun farming.[42] He built dormitories and kitchens for the orphans of the island, and by 1883 he was caring for forty-four children. He loved them, especially the ones who, like him, were poorly behaved. One leper, Joseph Manu, who had grown up in Damien's orphanage, recalled in the 1930s: "I was myself a naughty boy, and often Damien acted as if he would pull my ear or give me a kick, but immediately afterward he gave me candy. He behaved likewise with the other kids, but they were not as naughty as I was. That is why Damien loved me more, and he kept me alive for a long time."[43]

Even though Joseph clearly established himself as the family favorite despite steep competition from forty-three other children, Damien taught all the orphans to farm and cook and encouraged them to fall in love and marry when (or if) they grew to adulthood.[44]

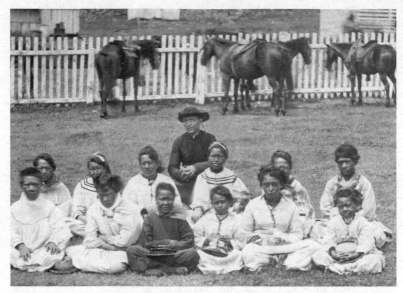

Look at this nineteenth-century Mr. Rogers.

He also did his best to break up what he regarded as vice on the island. The lepers had figured out that in addition to selling some of those sweet potatoes they were farming, they could also turn them into liquor. That sounds extremely enterprising and like the kind of brew you could sell for a *fortune* in Brooklyn right now. Damien, however, was not enthusiastic about this initiative. He often went to the area where drinkers would congregate—known as the "crazy pen"—armed with his walking stick. He used that stick to gesture, to whack people, and to break bottles of liquor. People fled as soon as they saw him coming.[45]

Righteous historians applaud these actions as a great idea, showing his commitment to virtue. But really that seems like a terrible way of curing people of their alcoholism. I think rehab consists of group counseling sessions and sharing feelings and not just "being attacked by a man carrying a large stick." But it was well intentioned. I'm sure if Damien were alive today, he would read the Big Book and choose a more appropriate method to counter alcoholism.

Although he was, clearly, not the kind of guy they could share a beer with, Damien did sit and have his nightly evening meal with the lepers. The group would sing songs, tell stories, drink tea, and Damien would share his pipe with them. Mealtime became known as "the time of peace between night and day."[46]

The sharing-his-pipe part might jump out at you here.

Leprosy isn't easily contracted, but Damien lived among the lepers so fully that he must have come to expect his fate many years before he actually developed the disease. I generally think that anyone who throws themselves in the path of a disease and doesn't take basic precautions is stupid and reckless. But . . . there was a little girl covered in worms because no one would change her bandages. What would you do?

The most common story about how Damien discovered he had leprosy is that one day in 1884 he was making a cup of tea for himself, or perhaps for someone else, at that time of peace between night and day. He spilled it, and the liquid ran down his foot. Anyone who has ever spilled scalding hot water on themselves will tell you that's a good time to leap, swear, and threaten legal proceedings against water manufacturers, but Damien felt nothing at all. Puzzled, he spilled more water upon his foot. Still nothing. The next day, he began his sermon not by saying, as he usually did, "My fellow believers" but by saying, as he would until the end of his life, "My fellow lepers." Contracting leprosy must have been terrifying, especially considering that Damien had always been so robust and active. But I hope he could have also looked around every day and seen the good that his life's work had wrought.

In 1888 when the English artist Edward Clifford visited the island, he wrote: "I had gone to Molokai expecting to find it scarcely less dreadful than hell itself, and the cheerful people, the lovely landscapes, and comparatively painless life were all surprises. These poor people seemed singularly happy." When Clifford asked the lepers *how* they could be so happy, they replied that they were doing fine, thanks, and "We like our pastor. He builds our houses himself, he gives us tea, biscuits, sugar and clothes. He takes good care of us and doesn't let us want for anything."[47] This was only a year before Damien died.

Damien remained active until the end, trying to build houses and care for his friends, and carving dolls for the children. He wrote to the bishop, who had asked him to come to Honolulu: "I cannot come for leprosy has attacked me. There are signs of it on my left cheek and ear, and my eyebrows are beginning to fall. I shall soon be quite disfigured. I have no doubt whatever about the nature of my illness, but I am calm and resigned and very happy in the midst of my people. I daily repeat from my heart, 'Thy will be done.'"[48] The bishop eventually persuaded him to be treated at the hospital in Honolulu. He was met by nuns, who were horrified to see that his face was now truly distorted and misshapen. Within two weeks, he was on a ship back to Molokai. On that voyage, the captain approached and asked if he could have a glass of wine with Damien. (He clearly hadn't heard about the walking stick.) Damien explained that would be unwise, because he was a leper, and common wisdom dictated you shouldn't drink with lepers. The ship captain replied that he understood, and he still wanted to, because he thought Damien was the bravest man he'd ever met.[49]

Damien died in 1889, shortly after his forty-ninth birthday. Just before his death he told the priest at his bedside, "If I have any credit with God, I shall intercede for all who are in the leproserie." The priest then asked if he could have Damien's mantle, hoping that with it, "[he] might inherit [Damien's] great heart." Damien laughed, rolled his eyes, and told him he couldn't because "it's full of leprosy."[50]

A pedestal erected on Molokai to the memory of Damien reads "Greater love hath no man than this, that a man lay down his life for his friends."[51] Damien deserves to be a saint, whether you think sainthood is proof of God's love for us or just a way to honor those who loved their fellow man.

No sooner had he, widely praised, died than some iconoclasts—or, as they are called today, mean jealous haters—appeared to disparage him. People are always going to have different opinions on public figures, even if they are the most perfect public figures in the history of the world. The Presbyterian minister C. M. Hyde wanted people to know that Damien was a *dirty slob* who *maybe had sex*. He wrote a letter to the *Sydney Presbyterian* on October 26, 1889, about Damien, stating:

> The simple truth is, he was a coarse, dirty man, headstrong and bigoted. He was not sent to Molokai, but went there without orders; did not stay at the leper settlement (before he became one himself), but circulated freely over the whole island (less than half the island is devoted to the lepers), and he came often to Honolulu. He had no hand in the reforms and improvements inaugurated, which were the work of our Board of Health, as occasion required and means were provided. He was not a pure man in his relations with women, and the leprosy of which he died should be attributed to his vices and carelessness.[52]

Most of that seems unfounded, and even if he was headstrong and careless, I'm on Damien's side. But I especially like the saints who are given to human vices, as are most of us. Of course that didn't stop people like Hyde—who, cool fact, was so paranoid about developing leprosy himself that he freaked out after using a Chinese laundry[53]—from disparaging him. The author Robert Louis Stevenson penned a lengthy defense of Damien's good deeds, to which Hyde responded by claiming that like other supporters of Damien, Stevenson was just a "bohemian crank, a negligible person, whose opinion is of no value to anyone."[54] Stevenson concluded the matter by stating, "Well, such is life."

Maybe I'm a bohemian crank too, but I don't think there is anyone in this book more heroic than Father Damien. He never confused the disease with the person suffering from it. He served as a role model to countless future heroes and heroines, most notably Mother Teresa, who specifically asked if he could be the saint for her congregation in 1984. At that time, he had not yet been canonized, as it was said that he had not performed miracles. Mother Teresa wrote to the pope claiming that she believed his two miracles were, first, "the removal of fear from the hearts of the lepers to acknowledge the disease and proclaim it and ask for medicine—and the birth of the hope of being cured." And second, the miraculous transformation of the community on Molokai to exhibit "greater concern, less fear, and readiness to help."[55]

However you feel about religion—because I do not want to get too *truly he followed in the footsteps of Christ* here—Damien is proof that kindness and love and compassion can be stronger forces than fear, even the fear of death. That's a good thing because we're all going to die. None of us can beat death. And so, perhaps, like Damien, we can go out into the world bravely and make it better for the time we are alive.

Individuals can change global perspectives on, well, just about anything. Before Damien's intercession people considered lepers barely human. I don't think Mother Teresa is overstating her case when she says that he performed a miracle in making people less afraid and more eager to fight against the miseries of the world.

In all likelihood, nobody reading this chapter is going to contract leprosy. A lot of the credit for that goes to Damien. He may not have found a cure—because not everyone's role is "being a doctor"—but his bravery raised awareness and inspired others to work for one. Not all of us can be expected to live up to

Damien's legacy, and not everyone needs to. There are lots of ways to help people on a smaller scale and without endangering your own health. But Damien is a reminder that you don't have to be a genius or a brilliant scientist or a doctor to help in this war against disease: you just have to be someone who gives a damn about your fellow man.

Typhoid

War is not an adventure.
War is disease. Like typhoid.

—ANTOINE DE SAINT-EXUPÉRY

If you take nothing else away from this book, I hope it's that sick people are not villains. They are unwell. It's impossible to say this enough. They should be sympathized with, instead of being declared sinners or degenerates or so many of the other negative labels society chooses to use. Diseases are villains and should be hunted down and combatted accordingly. Separating the disease from the diseased seems crucial if we are to be decent and compassionate people.

But having a disease doesn't necessarily make someone a good person. In certain cases diseased people do seem to lapse into villainy, and there's no more interesting example of this phenomenon than the story of Mary Mallon.

Mary Mallon's life in the United States was flourishing in 1907, perhaps going even better than her fellow Irish immigrants could have hoped for during that time period. She had come to

America as a teenager, and by the time she was thirty-seven, her superb cooking skills had earned her employment with an upper-crust family living on Park Avenue in New York City. She was earning around $45 a month. That would equate to $1,180 today, which may seem low but was a good salary for a cook at the time.[1]

Now, you might ask, especially if you are reading this chapter on your lunch break, what were Mary Mallon's specialties?

Desserts.

If you were a wealthy person in the late nineteenth/early twentieth century, desserts centered on ice cream. It had become especially popular following the publication of Agnes Marshall's two cookbooks about ice cream in 1885 and 1894.[2]

Mary Mallon was known for her peach melba, which is basically vanilla ice cream with peaches and raspberry sauce. It looks like a very healthy sundae with no sprinkles (because sprinkles were not invented until the 1930s). The summer of 1906 was a great time for peaches, according to the *Long Islander* newspaper, which reported "the largest and finest peaches that have been shown in town this season."[3] So Mary would have had the means to make a great deal of her specialty on a regular basis.

All of this could have been wonderful. Mary Mallon's story could be a nice account of an immigrant who made good in America by virtue of her cooking skills. It could be adapted by the Hallmark Channel, and people would watch it on National Ice Cream Day (the third Sunday in July). The close-up shots of Victorian/Edwardian ice cream would be *delightful.*

Unfortunately for Mary, her employers, and the producers at Hallmark, she was not well. Her body was teeming with *Salmonella typhii,* the bacteria that result in typhoid fever.[4] If people are infected with *Salmonella typhii,* their feces or, more rarely, their urine will contain the bacteria. That means that if they don't clean their hands thoroughly before preparing food, they might pass the bacteria on to the diners. Typhoid can also be spread by drinking water that's been contaminated by the bac-teria. Even eating shellfish from a polluted body of water could pass on the disease. At the turn of the century, if untreated, the disease resulted in death about 60 percent of the time. Today, antibiotics reduce the risk of fatality to almost zero.[5]

That said, typhoid fever is still prevalent in many periphery countries, and the Centers for Disease Control and Prevention (CDC) suggests that if you're in one of those locales you should "boil it (water), cook it (food), peel it (fruit), or forget it." Vacci-nations are also available. If you're traveling to a country where typhoid fever is still present, you should get a vaccination so your feeble little core country immune system does not expe-rience the extremely high fever (generally around 103 or 104 degrees, compared to the fever from the flu, which usually tops out at 101 degrees), headaches, muscle weakness, and diarrhea associated with the disease.

If you do not worry very much about contracting typhoid fever in your daily life, well, neither did wealthy people at the turn of the century. It was a disease associated with the urban poor, who, especially prior to the Tenement House Act of 1901, often lived in overcrowded and unsanitary conditions.

But the rich could contract typhoid if their food was handled by someone shedding *Salmonella typhii* bacteria. A cook could transfer those germs to the food *easily*. An investigator would later say, "I suppose no better way could be found for a cook to cleanse her hands of microbes and infect a family."[6] That wouldn't be so bad if the food was cooked. Cooking, as the CDC points out, will kill the bacteria. But on uncooked food—like ice cream— germs could slide into your intestines and thrive in their warm, moist environment. In the course of a day, a single bacterium cell can multiply into 8 million cells. They're just like beautiful little sea monkeys that way.

So would you hire a cook who appeared to have typhoid fever? Not unless you had a death wish. No one would hire a woman who was visibly ill to prepare their food. A woman who was ill with a temperature of 104 degrees probably wouldn't be able to prepare food to begin with. As long as everyone knew who made the food, and that person wasn't ill, everyone should be fine. Right?

Nope!

Here's the twist: Mary Mallon was an asymptomatic carrier of typhoid. Although she carried the bacteria inside her and could transmit it to others, she never suffered any of the symptoms herself. This is as close as someone can get to having a villainous superpower in real life.

But Mary didn't know she was spreading the disease. Yet considering the extent to which everyone around her contracted typhoid, she must have suspected she was at least very unlucky. Mary left a trail of illness wherever she went. The basic timeline of her employment goes like this:[7]

Summer 1900, Mamaroneck, New York: Mary worked for a family for three years and killed only one person. He was a visitor who became sick with typhoid about ten days after he arrived.

Winter, 1901–02, New York City: Mary infected a family's laundress during her eleven-month tenure.

Summer 1902, Dark Harbor, Maine: When Mary worked for the family of J. Coleman Drayton, seven of the nine members of the household (four members of the family, five servants) became ill, which led doctors to believe that . . . the footman did it. Really. As in a murder mystery where the characters think the butler is too obvious a suspect.

Summer 1904, Sands Point, New York: Four servants became sick. Doctors assumed that the laundress must have brought the disease.

Summer 1906, Oyster Bay, New York: Six of the eleven people in the Charles Henry Warren household became infected (three family members and three servants). This time people suspected the water supply might have been contaminated, and that the workers cleaning the water tank might have carried in the contagion on their boots.

Autumn 1906, Tuxedo Park, New York: A laundress became ill shortly after Mary arrived at the home of George Kessler.

Winter 1907, New York City: Mary began working at the Park Avenue home of Walter Brown. Two months after she was hired a maid became ill with typhoid, then the family's daughter contracted it and died.

Mary infected a total of twenty-two people. Is twenty-two a plague? No, of course not! It is approximately "an awful lot of people to have for Thanksgiving, too many, really" or "a manageable classroom size." The particular strain of the disease spread by Mary Mallon was not so widespread as to qualify as a plague. Indeed, in wealthy areas like Oyster Bay there seemed to be no other cases of infection beyond those in the house Mary occupied.[8]

That is not to say that, overall, typhoid itself isn't a plague. It still affects approximately 21.5 million people a year worldwide according to the CDC. The disease as it affected Mary and the people who came into contact with her is just one fascinating case of a much larger issue. But it's still the most fun to look at, as the outbreak surrounding Mary Mallon ties to some serious early twentieth-century sleuthing and tabloid journalism. And Sherlock Holmes–style investigating and sensational reporting were the best things about the 1900s. Those things and the non-typhoid ice cream.

The Sherlock Holmes figure in this case was a sanitation engineer named George A. Soper. The outbreak might never have been traced if the owners of the house in Oyster Bay—who had rented it to the Warrens in the summer of 1906—weren't concerned that they wouldn't be able to rent their house again. Accordingly, they were more diligent in investigating the root of the disease than the other affected families. They had every water source that might be contaminated tested. All of those tests came back negative. Stymied, they hired Soper, who had successfully investigated several typhoid outbreaks in the past.

Soper did not immediately think, *Probably the perfectly healthy cook caused the typhoid outbreak* because no one at the time would consider that possibility. He initially assumed the Warrens became ill because they were eating contaminated clams, which they routinely bought from a woman who lived in a tent and who found her catch in areas filled with sewage. But then he realized, "If clams had been responsible for the outbreak it did not seem clear why the fever should have been confined to this house. Soft clams form a very common article of diet among the native inhabitants of Oyster Bay."[9]

Apparently, everyone on Long Island ate probably polluted clams, which is awful. Well, for everyone except the tent woman, who was doing a brisk business with her sewage catch.

Soper knew that the first person in the Warren house who became sick fell ill on August 27, so he began looking for any significant changes to the family's situation just before then. He found that they had hired their new cook, Mary Mallon, on August 4, three weeks earlier. Soper understandably wanted to question her—perhaps to see if she had been serving anything more horrifying than clams fished out of sewage—but she had left the family three weeks after the typhoid outbreak. He began researching her employment history and found the unusually high instance of typhoid in each of the places she had worked.

By early March 1907 he found Mary at her new employer's Park Avenue address. He asked the healthy—indeed, robust— Mary to provide specimens so he could test to see if she had typhoid fever. The request honestly didn't entail all that much. Soper just needed to see if bacteria showed up in her urine, blood, or stool. On the whole, the process would have likely been less invasive than your annual physical. But Mary was *not* having it. And why should she? She was in perfect health, and the idea of being an asymptomatic carrier was barely known

within the medical community in 1907. She refused and forced
Soper from the house, furiously brandishing a carving fork at
him. Not deterred, Soper returned with a medical colleague,
and, again, Mary sent them away.[10]

So on March 11, 1907, Soper appealed to the New York
Health Department. He explained that he had not been able to
get Mary's consent to an examination, but that he believed "the
cook was a competent cause of typhoid and a menace to the
public health."[11] The department responded by sending an inspector named Dr. Sara Josephine Baker to visit Mary. Perhaps it
assumed the two might get along better because Dr. Baker was a
woman. It might have also thought, given that Baker had decided
to become a doctor after her father and brother died of typhoid
(despite her family's protestations that such a career choice was
an "unheard of, harebrained and unwomanly scheme"),[12] that
she would be able to convey to Mary the importance of protect-
ing other people from typhoid.

When Dr. Baker arrived, Mary attempted to stab her in the
neck, again with her trusty carving fork. Dr. Baker leaped back
into the hallway. She later wrote, "I learned afterward that Soper
had reason to suspect that Mary might make trouble, but I knew
nothing of that."[13] Mary fled. Dr. Baker called the police, who
helped her search the house. They found Mary in one of the closets.
Given that it took five hours to find her, one can only assume
none of them were great at playing hide-and-seek as children.
When Mary was discovered, Dr. Baker wrote, "She came out
fighting and swearing, both of which she could do with appalling efficiency and vigor."[14]

That Mary. She had spunk!

The police subdued her and took her to the Willard Parker
Hospital.[15] Dr. Baker claimed, "I sat on her all the way to the hospital. It was like being in a cage with an angry lion."[16] She would
later state, "The hardest dollars I ever earned were those as a

$100 a month Health Department employee when I was sent to get Mary Mallon."[17]

When Mary was finally tested at the hospital, doctors found that her stool was filled with typhoid bacteria. Her blood also tested positive for the disease.[18]

In an effort to isolate Mary, the health department moved her to a home on the Riverside Hospital grounds on North Brother Island, a small island in New York City's East River. Here, it suddenly becomes clear why Mary fought being taken away. She would be a virtual prisoner for the next three years. On North Brother Island Mary claimed that she was treated "like a leper" and that she had to live in an isolated house with only a dog for a companion.[19] Her abode was said to be either a "shack," a "pig-sty [with] a bad stench," or "a lonely little hut," depending upon the source.[20] None of those sounds good. While she was there she submitted 163 cultures, of which three-quarters tested positive for typhoid.[21] The fact that she definitely carried typhoid may have made the examiners feel justified in their treatment of Mary, but it did nothing to assuage her unhappiness. Later she would recall, "When I first came here I was so nervous and almost prostrated with grief and trouble. My eyes began to twitch, and the left eyelid became paralyzed and would not move. It remained in that condition for six months."[22] Despite the fact that there was an eye specialist on the island, he never visited Mary. She occupied some of her time writing letters to Soper and Dr. Baker, threatening to kill them when she got out, to which Dr. Baker noted, "I could not blame her for feeling that way."[23] Soper remarked, "She could write an excellent letter."[24]

In 1909 reporters at the *New York American* told the story of her situation, describing Mary Mallon as "Typhoid Mary." They wrote: "It is probable that Mary Mallon is a prisoner for life. And yet she has committed no crime, has never been accused of an immoral or wicked act, and has never been a prisoner in any court, nor has she been sentenced to imprisonment by any judge."[25] *Totally true.* Mary was quick to respond. In June 1909 she wrote a letter to the editor of the *New York American*, which was never published, explaining her frustration: "In reply to Dr. Park of the Board of Health I will state that I am not segregated with the typhoid patients. There is nobody on this island that has typhoid. There was never any effort by the Board authority to do anything for me excepting to cast me on the island and keep me a prisoner without being sick nor needing medical treatment."[26]

Were the doctors trying to cure her? Well, kind of. In addition to taking a ton of samples of her bodily functions, Mary claimed:

> [An authority] went to that doctor, and he said, "I cannot let that woman go, and all the people that she gave the typhoid to and so many deaths occurred in the families she was with." Dr. Studdiford said to this man, "Go and ask Mary Mallon and enveigle her to have an operation performed to have her gallbladder removed. I'll have the best surgeon in town to do the cutting." I said, "No. No knife will be put on me. I've nothing the matter with my gallbladder." Dr. Wilson asked me the very same question. I also told him no. Then he replied, "It might not do you any good." Also the supervising nurse asked me to have an operation performed. I also told her no, and she made the remark, "Would it not be better for you to have it done than remain here?" I told her no.[27]

If you've ever seen the television series *The Knick* (2014–present), you might also hesitate to have a doctor circa 1909 perform surgery on you, especially if you felt perfectly healthy. Mary went on: "I have been in fact a peep show for everybody. Even the interns had to come to see me and ask about the facts already

known to the whole wide world. The tuberculosis men would say
'There she is, the kidnapped woman.' Dr. Park has had me illustrated in Chicago. I wonder how the said Dr. William H. Park
would like to be insulted and put in the *Journal* and call him or
his wife Typhoid William Park."[28]

Despite their efforts and theories, there was actually very
little anyone could do to stop Mary from potentially infecting
others with typhoid. That theory that she'd be cured if only they
removed her gallbladder? Not so accurate. By 1914 Dr. Park concluded: "Medicinal treatment or surgery seems so far to have
yielded only slight results . . . Removal of the gall-bladder cannot
be relied upon."[29] It was becoming increasingly obvious that
isolating Mary for life was, at the very least, according to Dr. Park
himself, impractical. As early as 1908 he had discussed Mary's
case at a meeting of the American Medical Association and had
remarked:

> It seems to me that any attempt to isolate and treat on bacterio-
> logic examinations . . . is impracticable. When we consider
> that the presence of the bacilli in the feces of these persons
> is often only occasional, that numerous contact cases hav-
> ing never had typhoid fever would not come under suspi-
> cion, and finally, the impracticability of isolating for life so
> many persons, we are forced to consider isolation utterly
> impracticable, except as in the case of the cook already
> described, where conditions increase the danger to such a
> point that an attempt at some direct prevention becomes an
> essential.[30]

Dr. Park concluded his speech with a kind of "monsters are
among us, trying to get to our water supply" sentiment, claiming:
"We must, therefore, as before, turn to the more general methods of preventing infection, such as safeguarding our food and
water, not only chiefly when typhoid fever is present, but at all

times, for we now know that in every community, whether it be large or small, unsuspected typhoid bacilli carriers may always be present."[31] He could have phrased it in a less terrifying way, but it is a good idea to boil your water if it's not sanitized.

After her story became known, Mary Mallon decided to go to court. Good for Mary! Since as long as she was not preparing food, she posed little risk to anyone, her imprisonment seemed unreasonable. She found an attorney, who some people claimed was financed by William Randolph Hearst, the owner of the *New York American*, which had shared her story. The newspaper claimed that "some welathy [sic] New Yorkers" supported Mary Mallon in her effort to seek release after reading of her plight on June 20, 1909, in an article that moved them to "pity for the lone woman who has not a relative or a friend to whom she can turn."[32] Maybe that was the case. Maybe Hearst was just being a really nice guy. Or maybe he wanted to maintain close ties to Mary because updates on her story sold papers.

Her lawyer, George Francis O'Neill, filed a writ of habeas corpus in June 1909. This constitutional right guarantees that when citizens are detained against their will, they are entitled to legal judgment about their situation. Mary's case would be brought before the New York State Supreme Court. This doesn't seem unreasonable. Mary was correct that she was stripped of her rights. It is not that hyperbolic to say that she was kidnapped. And during this time other asymptomatic carriers had been found who were *not* detained. Mary even submitted to a lawyer samples of her feces that tested negative for typhoid.

Yet many people were, also understandably, concerned about the risk that carriers like Mary might pose to the public's health, and her release was a controversial topic at the time. This led to some exquisitely sarcastic solutions, such as the *New Thought Student*'s letter to the editor published in the *New York Times*:

If one unfortunate woman must be labeled "Typhoid Mary," why not send her other companions? Start a colony on some unpleasant island, call it "Uncle Sam's suspects," there collect Measles Sammy, Tonsillitis Joseph, Scarlet Fever Sally, Mumps Matilda, and Meningitis Matthew. Add Typhoid Mary, request the sterilized prayers of all religionized germ fanatics, and then leave the United States to enjoy the glorious freedom of the American flag under a medical monarchy.[33]

Anyhow, that's how the X-Men started.

If you are surprised that there was public outcry about an Irish immigrant (a member of a marginalized group at the time) being held against her will, well I'm with you. I didn't expect the public to be on Mary's side. This is an instance in history when people truly seemed to value "freedom for all" over "safety for some."

Despite the public support, the initial ruling in Mary's case did not improve her situation. In July 1909 it was decided that she was too dangerous to mingle with the public. The judge ruled that "the said petitioner, Mary Mallen [sic] be . . . hereby remanded to the custody of the Board of Health of the City of New York."[34]

But she wouldn't stay so for long. Almost immediately after the trial the newspaper coverage exploded, largely taking up Mary's cause. The public health official Charles Chapin stated, most likely in the Boston Transcript: "It seems a hardship to keep her virtually in prison, to deprive her of her liberty, because she happens to be the type of a class now known to be numerous and well distributed." He suggested instead: "There are many occupations in both city and country in which she could do little harm . . . there are hundreds of occupations in any one of which she might be free, but under a sort of medical probation."[35]

When Ernst J. Lederle was made the new Board of Health commissioner, he seemed to agree with Chapin. Lederle released

Mary in 1910 because, as he put it, "she has been shut up long enough to learn the precautions that she ought to take."[36]

Here are the actions the Board of Health took with Mary while she was at North Brother Island:

- Obtained many samples of her feces
- Offered to remove her gallbladder
- Gave her pills
- Allowed her to hang out with a dog and write murder threats

Here is an action they did not take:

- Teaching her a new job

Apparently, the board did not consider teaching her hygiene precautions or new job skills at North Brother Island. Where is a government-sponsored reeducation program when you need one?

Lederle, perhaps having some inkling of how this situation would play out, wondered upon Mary's release, "What will she do now? She is a good cook and until her detention had always made a comfortable living. I really do not know what she can do."[37] And then I imagine he exclaimed, "Well, I guess she'll figure it out!" and wandered off, whistling and chortling, "Remember, you're a good cook, Mary!"

I cannot stress enough how Mary should have been taught other job skills. Because, as I suspect everyone reading this chapter can guess, Mary went right on cooking. After 1912 she stopped reporting to the Board of Health. She began working under the pseudonym "Mrs. Brown." By 1915 she took a job in a place populated by babies with weak little immune systems.

That is a monstrous thing to do.

Dr. Sara Josephine Baker explains it more eloquently:

"Typhoid appeared in the Sloane Maternity Hospital in New York City, with two deaths out of twenty-five cases. Although I was no longer a roving inspector, I went up there one day and walked into the kitchen. Sure enough, there was Mary earning her living in the hospital kitchen and spreading typhoid germs among mothers and babies and doctors and nurses like a destroying angel."[38]

Mary was quarantined once more on North Brother Island. This time the public was far less sympathetic. Soper claimed: "Most persons will agree that no amount of dullness, anywhere this side of downright feeble-mindedness, can excuse [her return to cooking], and Mary Mallon is not feeble, either in mind or body. She is an excellent cook and has shown considerable ability in various other ways."[39]

On July 11, 1915, an article in the *Richmond Times-Dispatch* pondered the problem of "people who are fountains of germs, scattering disease and death all their lives—and the problem of what to do with them."[40] The article included an illustration depicting a cook casually tossing some skulls into a pan. The piece, written by John B. Huber, M.D., did an impressive job of fearmongering. People Huber claimed could be asymptomatic carriers of typhoid included your cook, dishwashers in hotels or restaurants or on ships, and any worker in a dairy. Pretty much anybody, really. However, he ended on a very sensible note: "It would not be necessary to confine typhoid carriers if they would only understand and observe the simple precautions they should take in order that the health and lives of others shall not be endangered by them. The activities of typhoid carriers must be so restricted that they shall never infect food nor their surroundings. In essence, all they have to do is be careful about their cleanliness."[41] He believed that the problem could be handled if people would simply "keep [their] hands clean . . . especially before handling food that others would have to eat."[42]

If you have ever wondered why you see those "Employees

Must Wash Hands" signs in restaurant bathrooms, well, here you go. Those signs are there so no one can Typhoid-Mary you.

But here's the thing people didn't understand at the time: Mary could not get her hands clean enough to prevent infecting anyone. If someone is shedding typhoid germs as Mary was, in order to have "clean" hands they have to wash them with soap for thirty seconds in 140-degree water. Water that hot causes third-degree burns within five seconds. You really just couldn't eat anything Mary prepared.[43]

Okay, she could have worn gloves. If all of this is making you very nervous, check that the guys preparing your burrito at Chipotle are wearing gloves. They almost invariably are, and also, they don't have typhoid fever.

The anxieties Mary Mallon induced linger on, even when people have forgotten their source. Most people today have no fear that individuals handling their food will give them typhoid. Most people today probably cannot describe exactly what typhoid entails. But a lot of them will still recoil at the thought of someone on a preparation line making their food without wearing gloves or restaurant employees failing to wash their hands.

One hundred years ago Huber's suggested protocols did not result in everyone just calmly washing their hands and practicing cleanliness. The idea that there were seemingly perfectly healthy people infecting others with deadly diseases simply by going about their daily business was *sensational* tabloid fodder. Journalists responded to outbreaks with a tone that bordered upon giddy delight. By August 22, 1920, the *Richmond Times-Dispatch* ran an article with the lengthy headline: "Mystery of the Poison Guest at Wealthy Mrs. Case's Party—Who Is the New 'Typhoid Mary' Who Haunted This Fashionable Society Function Like an Angel of Death, Scattering the Disease Germs That Made Thirty-Nine Women Seriously Ill and Have Already

Killed Two Victims?"[44] The article was accompanied by a picture of a skeleton wearing what appears to be a very pretty hat.

Stories like these would go on for years. In 1924 the baker Alphonse Cotils, an asymptomatic carrier, was "found preparing a strawberry pancake."[45] Then the confectioner Frederick Moersch infected twenty-eight people with his ice cream in 1928. People seemed as hungry for stories about these people as they had once been for the delicacies these men prepared. Unlike Mary, though, these people were treated more leniently and given suspended sentences in Cotils's case or allowed to stay at home in Moersch's.

Mary Mallon was confined for the rest of her life at North Brother Island. She began working at the Riverside Hospital as a helper. She supposedly enjoyed working in the laboratory, so it's a shame that those weren't skills she was taught earlier in life. She died of complications following a stroke at age seventy, on November 11, 1938.

Of Mary, Dr. Baker wrote:

> From my brief acquaintance with Mary, I learned to like her and to respect her point of view. After all, she has been of great service to humanity. There have been many typhoid carriers recognized since her time but she was the first charted case and for that distinction she paid in a life-long imprisonment. Today, typhoid carriers are usually allowed their freedom after they have pledged themselves not to handle other people's food. And, so far as we have been able to discover, they have kept their word. It was Mary's tragedy that she could not trust us.[46]

The government and the afflicted came to a place in this outbreak of disease where they both behaved sensibly and compassionately, and, at least by Dr. Baker's account, with some exceptions, that approach *worked*. Of course, on both sides, cooperation requires a sizable degree of trust. People have to be able to trust officials to see them as individuals, not just as a transport system for a disease. They also have to trust that officials will not lie to them when told they are ill, even if they don't feel sick. The government, in turn, has to trust that people will not go out of their way to harm their fellow citizens. All of that trust seems very much a matter of faith, but it's not impossible to achieve. It just requires everyone not being the absolute worst.

Spanish Flu

Influenza, labeled Spanish, came and beat
me to my knees;
Even doctors couldn't banish from my form
that punk disease.

—WALT MASON

The purpose of this book is not to scare you. Instead, like all good books, it is intended to distract you from the screaming baby one aisle over from the airplane seat where you are currently trapped for the next five hours. So I apologize that I have to tell you to smile at the frazzled parent, put on your earphones, and brace yourself, because about one hundred years ago, in 1918, 50 million people worldwide died of the Spanish flu, and we still don't know what caused it or how to treat it, how to eradicate it, or if it will ever return. Sorry!

We do know that this disease wasn't Spanish. In all likelihood, the Spanish flu was an all-American plague hailing from Haskell, Kansas. There is still research that attempts to pin the biggest plague in the twentieth century on anyplace else (guesses range from China to Great Britain), probably because "America's bread-basket" is a much nicer way to refer to the Midwest than "the planet's flu bin."

In spite of our First World desire to believe that diseases are fundamentally exotic imports, the first case of the Spanish flu epidemic was reported to the weekly journal *Public Health Reports* by Dr. Loring Miner of Haskell, Kansas, in March 1918. Since the early winter, Dr. Miner had been shocked to see dozens of his patients become sick with what seemed to be "influenza of a severe type" and die. They weren't even older, less robust patients. The deceased were people who seemed to be extremely healthy and in the prime of life. When Dr. Miner called the U.S. Public Health Service to describe his unusual findings, it wasn't able to offer any help. Despite his notice in *Public Health Reports*, people didn't seem to take the outbreak all that seriously.[1]

This might be a good time to mention that if you learn about an airborne virus that seems to be killing otherwise healthy young people in your area from a reputable medical journal, you are reading very bad news. Go to the grocery store and start stocking up on supplies *immediately*. If you have someplace relatively isolated to live, go there. Doing so might feel a bit silly or paranoid, but, honestly, neither of those responses would be overreactions.

Of course, at the time, no one followed Loring's sage advice. People may have been cavalier because almost everyone has had the flu once and survived. During the early 1900s there was even a jokey doctor's saying about influenza that went, "Quite a godsend! Everybody ill, nobody dying."[2] Even today, if you mention Spanish flu, most will think that maybe some people had to take a week or two off work in Spain because they were throwing up a whole lot. Because, sure, the flu is inconvenient, but it's something most people are able to survive.

This wasn't that sort of flu. Dr. Miner was describing a disease that was deadliest in the healthiest people, adults between the ages of twenty-five and twenty-nine.[3] The historian Dr. Alfred Crosby explained this phenomenon on the PBS TV series *American Experience*: "One of the factors that made this so particularly frightening was that everybody had a preconception of what the flu was: it's a miserable cold and, after a few days, you're up and around. This was a flu that put people into bed as if they'd been hit with a two-by-four. That turned into pneumonia, that turned people blue and black and killed them. It was a flu out of some sort of a horror story."[4]

One of the good things about flu, however, is that it burns out pretty fast. Haskell was a relatively isolated town. At any other time—other than now, obviously, when people probably catch a plane to New York from Kansas without thinking about it—the illness might have stopped right there. But in 1918 large numbers of young men from the area were traveling to a military camp to train for battle in World War I.[5]

Camp Funston, also in Kansas (it was an encampment of Fort Riley), housed twenty-six thousand young soldiers, making it the second-largest training camp in the country. So it was the second-worst place for a young man sick with a superdeadly strain of young-people-killing flu to go. Especially because that winter the "barracks and tents were overcrowded," which meant that men hung out in close, cramped proximity to one another.[6] March 4 brought the first report of someone at Funston becoming sick with what seemed to be a severe type of influenza. Within three weeks, 1,100 men at the camp had the flu and 38 had died.[7]

That's not a shocking percentage, unless you consider the fact that no one expected healthy twenty-year-olds to die of the flu at all. A table in Dr. Crosby's book *America's Forgotten Pandemic: The Influenza of 1918* shows that in 1917 flu deaths were highest—around 30 to 35 percent of those contracting the disease—among babies and those over age sixty. (Don't worry, older readers. Age sixty then is probably like being over age ninety today.) People outside of those age groups died of flu less than 10 percent of the time. So the chart of age and flu death usually looks like a *U*. Meanwhile, the chart of influenza deaths in 1918 looked like a crazy, badly drawn *N*. Around 20 percent of affected babies seemed to die, followed by a drop down to the standard less than 10 percent, followed by a spike in deaths beginning at age nineteen, and returning to normal levels by around middle age. By 1918, 35 percent of people dying from influenza were in their twenties.

Apparently, the disease overstimulated healthy immune systems, turning them against the body. In slightly more medical terms, the Spanish flu triggered what's called a *cytokine storm*. Cytokine proteins exist in your body to modulate the release of immune cells when there is an infection. A healthy immune system has a lot of those little fellows. In a cytokine storm, too many immune cells flood the site of the infection, which causes inflammation around that site. If the site of the infection is in the lungs—as it could be in a respiratory disease like the Spanish flu—the inflamed lungs fill with fluids. Then you die.[8]

You would think that if there was a strange new disease killing young soldiers, everyone would be reading about it everywhere. Remember the recent ebola outbreak, which killed a grand total of two people in the United States? That dominated the American news cycle for months.

So it seems insane that a disease killing young heterosexual white men in the middle of America would just be overlooked. (I'm not saying that diseases affecting other groups should be ignored; simply that, historically, they have been.) Were newspaper reporters really dense one hundred years ago? No. They didn't report on the outbreak because they did not want to go to jail.

A morale law had been passed in 1917 after the United States entered World War I. It stated you could receive twenty years in jail if you chose to "utter, print, write or publish any disloyal, profane, scurrilous, or abusive language about the government of the United States."[9] This law seems unconstitutional, but it was upheld by the Supreme Court ruling (*Schenck v. United States*) that you can't say things that "represent to society a clear and present danger." So you cannot scream "Fire!" in a crowded theater, and you can't say that a terrifying disease is spreading through the populace and the government has no idea how to combat it.

The difference between the two is that the first one presupposes a fire does not actually exist. If there is a blaze in a crowded theater, you should still scream "Fire!" You should scream it loudly. People need to know so they can make decisions about what to do. An even better option would be to scream, "Fire! The exits are clearly lit! Proceed to them!" (You are an usher in this situation.) Similarly, you should also loudly let people know about the terrifying new disease sweeping through the country, hopefully with some helpful thoughts on how to proceed in the face of such a menace.

But American reporters really didn't want to risk those twenty years of jail time.

The press in Britain was even more severely censored during World War I. There, the Defense of the Realm Act declared, "No person shall by word of mouth or in writing spread reports likely to cause disaffection or alarm among any of His Majesty's forces or among the civilian population."[10] In Britain, "journalistic outlaws" were threatened with execution.

Newspapers in the United States were supposed to present the truth, but they were also supposed to report cheerful facts that made America look good. Whenever someone jaded by today's news tells you that they want a newspaper that just shares *good* news, remind them that President Woodrow Wilson tried that approach. It did not work out so well. The writer Walter Lippmann, who—cool fact—later came up with the phrase *Cold*

War, urged the president to create a publicity bureau that would publish only articles favorable to the United States. That is because Lippmann believed that most citizens were "mentally children or barbarians." Wilson founded the department one day after receiving Lippmann's memo, appointing George Creel to run it. The Committee on Public Information went on to distribute tens of thousands of articles about America's greatness, which newspapers ran largely unedited. After all, given that editors were fearful of publishing anything that might be construed as anti-American, they were happy for some additional articles to fill up pages.[11]

Lippmann may have viewed the populace as children, but even kids were able to figure out what was going on with the flu. Before long, they had begun singing a schoolyard rhyme that went:

> *I had a little bird,*
> *Its name was Enza.*
> *I opened the window*
> *and in flew Enza.*

The Spanish flu worked fast. The epidemiologist Shirley Fannin reported: "If an individual with influenza were standing in front of a room full of people coughing, each cough would carry millions of particles with disease-causing organisms into the air. All the people breathing that air would have an opportunity to inhale a disease-causing organism. It doesn't take very long for one case to become 10,000 cases."[12]

The disease started moving with the soldiers to other army camps around the country and then overseas. People could be infected and then die within twenty-four hours. However, news reports, where they existed at all in the American media, insisted that everything was fine. That was more or less what they would keep reporting—ridiculous though it increasingly seemed—through the entirety of the epidemic.

Spain, however, was neutral during World War I. That meant the Spanish press could report on the flu and its growing number of fatalities without fear of being jailed or labeled unpatriotic. On May 22, 1918, Spanish newspapers ran an article about a new kind of illness that seemed to be sickening many citizens. Since May is a month with numerous festivals, at first it was thought the disease might be foodborne, as entire parties of people fell ill. By May 28, King Alfonso of Spain was sick. So were a staggering 8 million other Spaniards.[13]

By July, influenza had made its way to London, where in the first week it killed 287 people.[14] In spite of this, English newspapers still claimed the disease was just "the general weakness of nerve-power known as war-weariness."[15] They were also skeptical of the spread of the disease in Spain. The *British Journal of Medicine* reported that influenza "appears to have been particularly widespread in Spain during the month of May; that there were 8 million cases of the disease in that country, as it was alleged by the French press at the time, is a statement requiring perhaps a grain of salt for deglutition, but certainly pointing to a very heavy incidence."[16] Look, that 8 million number might be overstated. We have no way of knowing. But we do know you should take newspapers trying to keep morale up during wartime with a whole canister of salt. The British army would carry that world weariness, or, as it later came to be called, "the Big Sneeze,"[17] all over the globe, and cases were soon turning up in India and North Africa.[18]

By fall, conditions were worse. In John M. Barry's words in *The Great Influenza*, the spread of the disease among so many people had turned it into "a better and more efficient killer." The autumn of 1918 is often considered to be the "second wave" of the disease.[19]

As the outbreak grew more deadly, more American troops were needed overseas. That was at least in part because in some units up to 80 percent of the men had died of Spanish flu. Dr. Victor Vaughn, the former president of the American Medical Association, stated, "This infection, like war, kills the young, vigorous, robust adults. The husky male either made a speedy and rather abrupt recovery or was likely to die."[20] Soldiers traveled to Europe on troop ships. In those crowded conditions, anyone who had the disease would certainly pass it on to others. When President Woodrow Wilson agreed that more young soldiers—men who would be at the most likely age to die of the disease—would have to be sent overseas (around 250,000 in October),[21] he reportedly turned to his aide and remarked, "I wonder if you have heard this limerick? 'I had a little bird and his name was Enza . . .' "[22]

Hearing this, do you think Woodrow Wilson a monster? Because he seems to be doing a very good imitation of Donald Sutherland's character in the movie trilogy *The Hunger Games* (2012–15). I'll actually spoil that for you and say, at the very least, Wilson had moral failings as large as the moon. He believed that immigrants to the United States represented "sordid and hapless elements of their population."[23] He literally kept African Americans in cages when they had to work on the same floor as white people because he didn't want them mingling (much to the outrage of their coworkers, some of whom they had worked with for decades). The civil rights leader W. E. B. Du Bois wrote to him about his general belief that "segregation was not humiliating but a benefit," and, specifically, about his forcible attempts to segregate people of different colors from working together, asking, "Do you know that no other group of American citizens has ever been treated in this way and that no President of the United States ever dared to propose such treatment?"[24] President Wilson, like Lippmann, fundamentally believed that all Americans were not equal. That surely made the idea of restricting the flow of information available to all Americans much more palatable.

So, yes, Wilson was not a good guy. Whether you find his decision regarding soldiers' deployment justifiable—and it seems like a fun theoretical situation to consider—depends on whether you think winning World War I was worth it at any cost.

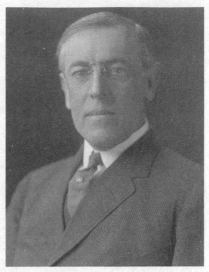

Also, his face looked like a rich man's pet bird.

Whoever takes on this project should keep in mind that Woodrow Wilson himself later contracted what is largely believed to be the Spanish flu, which prevented him from engaging fully in the Treaty of Versailles peace talks, the terms of which are often said to have so deeply penalized Germany that they led to World War II.[25]

Whatever your opinion of Wilson at this moment (he's awful), we have the advantage of looking at his actions from a hundred years in the future. He was focused on the war at hand.

Everyone was focused on the war at hand.

It is almost impossible, living as we do in a time without morale laws, to imagine how glorious World War I was considered to be by the American people. Patriotism was so high that young men would have been clamoring to get on the troop ship. The culture was suffused with references to how great it was to go fight the Hun. Immensely popular songs like "Over There" encouraged young men to

Hurry right away, no delay, go today
Make your daddy glad to have had such a lad
Tell your sweetheart not to pine
to be proud her boy's in line.[26]

while women at home would chant,

Tramp, tramp, tramp the boys are marching.
I spy Kaiser at the door.
And we'll get a lemon pie and we'll squash him in his eye
and there won't be any Kaiser anymore.[27]

It seems the men got the better song. That lemon pie ditty was like a child's take on how to end fascism if that child was also obsessed with Charlie Chaplin and baked goods. If you hit someone with a pie, that person just doesn't *disappear*. If that were true, there would be no clowns.

As enthusiastic as men might have been about participating in the war, they probably would have been less enthused about the prospect of dying from flu on a ship. But newspapers weren't going to tell them about that. The government wasn't going to, either. Officials claimed that they had everything under control and that the soldiers and the populace had nothing to worry about. Royal Copeland, the health commissioner in New York, claimed, "You haven't heard of our doughboys getting it, have you? You bet you haven't, and you won't . . . No need for our people to worry over the matter."[28]

You *should* have heard about it. During World War I, forty thousand American soldiers were killed by Spanish flu. For perspective, that's only seven thousand fewer American soldiers than were killed in combat in Vietnam. Dr. Vaughn later remarked, "The saddest part of my life was when I witnessed the hundreds of deaths of the soldiers in the Army camps and did not know what to do. At that moment I decided never again to prate about the great achievements of medical science and to humbly admit our dense ignorance in this case."[29]

Hushing up the epidemic took more and more work by the press. As late as September 26, headlines in the *El Paso Herald* proclaimed "Vicious Rumors of Influenza Epidemic Will Be Combatted," while sailors were told to write home and tell their relatives not to worry about the stories spreading about the disease.[30]

Meanwhile, in Philadelphia—one of the largest and most overcrowded cities in the United States at the time—the disease began to present among members of the navy gathering there in early September. By September 15, six hundred navy men were in the hospital. The navy hospital was overflowing. The sick had to be sent to civilian hospitals, where they would begin spreading the disease farther.

This would have been a great time for officials to *adamantly* start advising people to stay inside. Or maybe not move people with a highly contagious disease to a hospital where people with other ailments would be. We can all play "How many better solutions can we find to this situation than a massive cover-up?"

The answer is "a lot."

However, officials in Philadelphia opted for the "massive cover-up" option. They continued to downplay the threat. The Board of Health advised people to keep warm, keep their feet dry, and avoid crowds. Perhaps if they had stressed the actual danger, Philadelphians wouldn't have ignored that "avoid crowds" message. Surely, hundreds of thousands of them wouldn't have come together for the Liberty Loan parade on September 28. Dr. Howard Anders—a public health expert who should stand out as one of the heroes in this book—begged a series of reporters to write about the danger posed by the parade. He had already written to the navy surgeon general, asking him to send in federal authorities to "insist upon safeguarding its men and, collaterally, the whole population of Philadelphia,"[31] to no avail.

He was correctly certain that congregating for a parade would spread influenza to thousands of civilians. All the newspapers refused his request—despite his description of the parade as "a ready-made inflammable mass for a conflagration," which is a fancy way of saying that this disease would *burn Philadelphia to the ground*—because they didn't want to hurt morale.[32]

None of those newspapers can be heroes in this book. Dr. Anders can. You may say, "Wait. He tried, but he did not succeed! There are no points for trying! Do or do not, there is no try!" To which I will say, "No, that's silly. The world is not dictated by Yoda's quips. Yoda is just a little monster who lives in a backpack. Of course there are points for trying." Dr. Anders tried to warn people, and that was more than anyone else was doing. He did the right thing, at a time when it was certainly easier to stay silent. This is my book, and I say he is a hero for trying.

He did fail, though.

I hope that parade was fun, because its consequences were every bit as devastating as Dr. Anders predicted. At the end of September, the director of the Philadelphia Department of Public Health and Charities, Dr. Wilmer Krusen, noted, "The epidemic is now present in the civilian population." This admission was a step in the right direction, so good work, Dr. Krusen. Unfortunately, by the time he finally spoke, hundreds of people were dying a day. Literally. On October 1, 117 people died of Spanish flu in Philadelphia. Still, on October 6, the *Philadelphia Inquirer* peppily reported that the best way to avoid the disease was to:

> Live a clean life.
> Do not even discuss influenza . . .
> Worry is useless.
> Talk of cheerful things instead of the disease.[33]

The newspaper went on to lament the very basic precautions of closing public gathering places like churches and movie theaters.[34] The *Inquirer* asked on October 6, "What are the authorities trying to do? Scare everyone to death?"[35] A blasé attitude, clean living, and cheerful thoughts didn't stop the disease. On October 10, 759 people died.[36]

There was a weird period during the fall months when everyone seemed to know about the disease, but no one seemed to take it very seriously. In Katherine Anne Porter's short story "Pale Horse, Pale Rider," there is a scene in which the protagonist, a theater critic, is welcoming her love interest, a soldier who is temporarily home on leave. It runs:

> "I wonder," said Miranda, "How did you manage to get an extension of leave?"
>
> "They just gave it," said Adam, "For no reason. The men are dying like flies out there, anyway. This funny new disease. Simply knocks you into a cocked hat."
>
> "It seems to be a plague," said Miranda, "something out of the middle ages. Did you see so many funerals, ever?"
>
> "Never did. Well, let's be strong minded and not have any of it . . . What a job you've got," said Adam, "nothing to do but run from one dizzy amusement to another and then write a piece about it."
>
> "Yes, it's too dizzy for words," said Miranda. They stood while a funeral passed, and this time they watched it in silence.[37]

Despite death surrounding them, the fact that they could be affected by the disease still seemed to shock people, as it did the characters in Porter's work. There was a decided focus on going about day-to-day business, cheerfully. Among the scant public health warnings about the Spanish flu were paper flyers that explained, "When obliged to cough or sneeze, always place a handkerchief, paper napkin, or fabric of some kind before the face."[38] This is good advice *if you have a cold.* A hanky is woefully insufficient to combat a highly infectious, deadly, airborne disease. Still, the headline on October 15 in the *Inquirer* cheerfully announced on one of its back pages, "Scientific Nursing Halting Epidemic . . . Officials Say Entire Situation Is Well in Hand."[39] That was not true. Despite the noble efforts of the nurses and physicians at the hospitals—and the nuns and various other volunteers who were working tirelessly—they were absolutely not halting the epidemic. They couldn't even respond to all the people who needed hospitalization.[40]

Horse-drawn carriages rolled through the streets of Philadelphia collecting dead bodies that had been rotting on the sidewalks. Why, you might understandably ask, have we suddenly been transported back to the fourteenth century? Likely because, as is usually the case when pandemics strike, coffins were in such high demand that they had become expensive. People had taken to stealing them. Children's corpses were stuffed into macaroni boxes. Yes, macaroni boxes used to be bigger, and no, the government clearly wasn't subsidizing funerals, because Woodrow Wilson wasn't as smart as Marcus Aurelius.[41] Even if you could procure a coffin, undertakers wouldn't touch dead bodies, so families had to bury their loved ones themselves. That is, if there was anyone healthy enough to do the burying. Philadelphia's citizenry were left waiting on their porches for a charity corpse truck, driven by priests, to come and collect their dead. You would have seen open trucks filled with dead bodies driving through the streets.[42] Those trucks would make a lot of rounds that month, because eleven thousand people died in Philadelphia that October.[43]

In Chicago, where the health commissioner claimed he'd "do nothing to interfere with the morale of the community" as "fear kills more than disease," the death rate climbed from

15 percent of the afflicted to 40 percent that same month.[44] As someone who is afraid of literally everything, I can assure you that fear does not have such a successful kill rate. In Buffalo, the acting city health commissioner claimed that "it was no uncommon matter to find persons who had waited two or three days after having repeatedly phoned or summoned physicians, suffering and dying because every physician was worked beyond human endurance."[45] Sophomores in medical school were called upon—well before they were properly trained physicians—to care for the afflicted. In New York City, 30,736 people died in September and October.[46] One doctor, at New York's Presbyterian Hospital, recalled going into the wards each morning and finding that every single patient in critical care had died. *Every morning.*[47]

All the doctors who worked through this epidemic and everyone who volunteered? They are heroes, too. The fact that they were not all awarded presidential medals for their service is an oversight.

Eventually, without clear guidance on what to do to effectively combat the disease and death, morale eroded. When people, who by this time were surrounded by clear evidence of the danger, attempted to find helpful information, they were met, over and over, with the message that everything was fine. Even when newspapers did offer truthful information, people were now unsure whether they could trust anything that was printed.

That October—which was the deadliest month in U.S. history, and that takes into account periods like, say, the Civil War—195,000 people died of the Spanish flu.[48] If you are in a house with anyone else right now, you can put this in perspective by shouting, "One us would be dead, probably!" Your family members love it when you do that. Now imagine Dr. Krusen in the background desperately exclaiming, as he did, "Don't get frightened or panic-stricken over exaggerated reports."[49] The newspapers printed admonitions that read, "Don't Get Scared." After the children's little bird poem, this may be the second-scariest, supposedly anodyne phrase in this chapter.

People were terrified.

In response, they began to behave like terrified people. They made placards that read, "Spitting Equals Death," and culprits began to be arrested for spitting.[50] I mean, that was not wrong (don't spit on people if you have the flu), but arresting people for bodily functions is not a way to calm panic, nor was it especially effective. Face masks became mandatory for civil servants and those suffering from influenza, though the *Washington Times* claimed that "it [was] not thought the use of masks will become general, and health officials inclined to doubt their value for general use as a preventative measure."[51] This announcement was far less prominent in the paper than the anticipatory exclamation "Thanksgiving Is Coming!" which was illustrated with a picture of a soldier running after a turkey who is wearing a fez, like the guy in the other kind of Turkey. Thanksgiving would not be coming for over a month.

Soon masks were in widespread use by ordinary citizens, but, sadly, officials were correct in their predictions that they didn't seem especially effective in combatting the disease.[52] People began to rely on outdated folk remedies like onions—just as they had in the times of the bubonic plague.[53] One shop merchant claimed he sold more quinine in one day than he had in the past three years, which would have been awesome and useful if only this had been an epidemic of malaria. Beyond quinine,[54] advertisements for influenza remedies included:

- Use Oil of Hyomei. Bathe your breathing organs with antiseptic balsam.
- Munyon's Paw Paw Pills for influenza insurance.
- Sick with influenza? Use Ely's Cream Balm. No more snuffling. No struggling for breath.[55]

(Paw paw pills sound like something that should treat a cat's ringworm.)

And it wasn't just superstitious people who took to dubious medical treatments. Doctors recommended consuming *more* alcohol—whiskey, half a bottle of wine a day, and a glass of port before bed.[56] Doctors started filling prescriptions for whiskey, which could be procured from drugstores in Philadelphia.[57] In most cases drinking doesn't solve anything, but in this particular instance *not* drinking wasn't helping—nothing was—so it may have been an understandable response.

In Philadelphia most popular gathering places were shut down, though not, officials stressed, as a public safety measure. However, suppressing information about the reasons for these closures led to great inefficiencies and much confusion. For instance, rather than telling people they should *really* avoid cramming together on streetcars, especially if they were feeling ill, officials just issued a limitation on the number of people who could be on streetcars at any time. A man in England claimed that his movie theater was safe—and he was believed—because he had a special aerating machine. He may have had such a machine, and he may very well have believed it was effective, but it was not.[58] Bars were the last establishments to close in Philadelphia,[59] but the Savoy Hotel in London did a brisk business with its new Corpse Reviver cocktail of whiskey and rum. (It was slightly different from the traditional hangover cure, but both are similar in their abilities to make people feel a little less like they are dying.)[60]

People began to take matters into their own, often panicked and sometimes inebriated, hands. A health inspector in San Francisco shot a man who refused to wear a mask, and a man in Chicago is said to have screamed, "I'll cure them my own way!" as he slashed open the throats of his family members.[61] In London another man similarly cut the throats of his wife and two daughters when he recognized that he'd contracted the disease and that they would be left poor after his death.[62]

Spanish influenza came to be referred to as "the plague," as in the bubonic plague of the fourteenth century. That can't be surprising. Despite the six hundred years that had passed, every aspect of the public disarray and nightmarish nature of this time was more reminiscent of the black death than of any other outbreak. An internal American Red Cross memo wrote that "a fear and panic of the influenza, akin to the terror of the middle ages regarding the Black Plague, has been prevalent in many parts of the country."[63] A Red Cross report in rural Kentucky explained that people had begun starving to death because they wouldn't venture outside for food.

By November it seemed that people had given up attempting to fight. They stayed at home, terrified. While earlier during the outbreak in New York, Lillian Wald, the nurse and humanitarian, spotted "dignified and discerning women [who] stood on the steps at Altman's and Tiffany's Fifth Avenue shops and accosted passers-by" hoping to get funds to help fight the epidemic, now no one seemed to want to go anywhere.[64] Elizabeth Martin, the head of Emergency Aid in Philadelphia, furiously reported that "hundreds of women who are content to sit back . . . had delightful dreams of themselves in the roles of angels of mercy, had the unfathomable vanity to imagine that they were capable of great spirit of sacrifice. Nothing seems to rouse them now. They have been told that there are families in which every member is ill, in which the children are actually starving because there is no one to give them food. The death rate is so high and they still hold back."[65] Dr. Victor Vaughn remarked: "If the epidemic continues its mathematical rate of acceleration, civilization could easily disappear from the face of the earth."[66] But, miraculously, it didn't.

We don't know precisely why the disease stopped killing people—scientists have various theories—but it did. The most common one is that it simply killed too many hosts.

It was only after it had abated—and after the war had

ended—that people began writing about it. The *American Journal of Medicine* stated on December 28, 1918:

> The year 1918 has gone: a year momentous as the termination of the most cruel war in the annals of the human race; a year which marked, the end at least for a time, of man's destruction of man; unfortunately a year in which developed a most fatal infectious disease causing the death of hundreds of thousands of human beings. Medical science for four and one-half years devoted itself to putting men on the firing line and keeping them there. Now it must turn with its whole might to combating the greatest enemy of all—infectious disease.[67]

But there was little to combat. While a milder third wave of the disease appeared the next winter—and there would be periodic outbreaks through the 1920s—the deadliest period was over.

The Spanish flu is estimated to have killed somewhere between 25 million and 100 million people over the world. Around 675,000 Americans are thought to have died of it. That's more than died in the Civil War, and the Civil War went on for four years.

Scientists today are experimenting with reverse genetics to try to re-create the flu, using virus that was preserved in frozen corpses. The hope is that they can develop a vaccine that would stop the disease if it emerges again. However, that's extremely challenging given the speed with which the virus has been known to mutate. They haven't succeeded yet.[68]

So the disease is still out there, perhaps lurking under the ice somewhere, and there's no cure.

If there's another outbreak, mankind might not be so lucky as to survive. But we can at least avoid being so stupidly duplicitous.

John Barry, in *The Great Influenza*, writes: "Those in authority must retain the public's trust. The way to do that is to distort nothing, to put the best face on nothing, to try to manipulate no one . . . Leadership must make whatever horror exists concrete. Only then will people be able to break it apart."[69]

There are certainly better ways for government officials to combat public health crises. Maybe at minimum they should subsidize funerals so no one has to bury their children in macaroni boxes. Planning for emergency response teams and finding volunteers early might also be a good strategy. Government leaders failed here, in just about every way they could fail, but, as terrible as Woodrow Wilson was, I am willing to admit he did have some other issues going on at the time.

It's the journalists I am most disappointed in. Perhaps because, ideally, journalists safeguard the public by telling them what they need to know. There's a trope in movies and books where a reporter at some point screams something like, "We're journalists! We tell the truth!" Sometimes that translates into some silly stuff, like honestly reporting to the public that Kim Kardashian has cellulite. But at its best, say, during Watergate or during the clergy abuse scandal, reporting the truth means that journalists act as public watchdogs. Often they defend the common man despite the wishes of those in power. They tell the truth, even when it would be easier to lie—when the government *wants* them to lie. That's the highest possible aim of the fourth estate. Sadly, Senator Hiram Johnson's 1917 claim that "the first casualty when the war comes is truth" proved accurate in this instance. In 1918, during the Spanish flu outbreak, owing to whatever misguided intentions, the fourth estate failed.

And although better coverage of the outbreak's evolution in the press couldn't have stopped the influenza virus, a single newspaper headline in Philadelphia saying "Don't Go to Any Parades; for the Love of God Cancel Your Stupid Parade" could have saved hundreds of lives. It would have done a lot more than those telling people, "Don't Get Scared!"

Telling people that things are fine is not the same as making them fine.

This failure is in the past. Journalists and editors had their reasons. Risking jail time is no joke. But learning from this breakdown in truth-telling is important because the fourth estate can't fail again. We are fortunate today to have organizations like the Centers for Disease Control and Prevention and the World Health Organization that track how diseases are progressing and report these findings. In the event of an outbreak similar to the Spanish flu, they will be wonderful resources. I hope we'll be similarly lucky to have journalists who will be able to share necessary information with the public. The public is at its strongest when it is well informed. Despite Lippmann's claims to the contrary, we are smart, and we are good, and we are always stronger when we work together. If there is a next time, it would be very much to our benefit to remember that.

Encephalitis Lethargica

*Only at times the curtain of the
pupils lifts, quietly—an image enters
in, rushes down through the tensed,
arrested muscles, plunges into the
heart and is gone.*

—Rainier Maria Rilke,
translated by Stephen Mitchel

Here is a graphic showing the pace of medical advances for most of our known history:

It is a line showing conditions improving really, really slowly until 1900. It is my totally accurate and scientific portrayal of every single step forward and setback. I had to look up how to draw in Microsoft Word, and it took me probably four minutes to learn how to make this line, so, please, take a second to appreciate it.

Here is what happens to medical progress in the twentieth century:

"Wow! Those are some finely drawn lines," you are probably saying. "It certainly seems as if we have made rapid advances in the last hundred years! But I want to see an even steeper line. Perhaps illustrating medical methods and treatments becoming radically more advanced within a single human lifetime. A fifty-year period or so. Accomplished drawer of lines—has such an event ever occurred?"

Do I have one such example for you! It is encephalitis lethargica—often abbreviated to EL—which raged from 1916 through the late 1920s. If you managed to get through the Spanish flu chapter and were only modestly terrified, well, you're a strange human being, but settle in and prepare to have your socks scared off. EL gives Spanish flu a run for its money in terms of "terrifying uncured diseases that we have forgotten about in less than one hundred years."

During the period in the teens and 1920s when EL was rampant, there were a million cases of the disease and more than five hundred thousand deaths worldwide.[1] Those who survived were often trapped inside their own bodies. It's a bit of a simplification, but you could think of it as a disease that turned you into a human statue, as in *A Winter's Tale*. For a slightly more clinical explanation, H. F. Smith, who worked for the U.S. Public Health Service, described the disease in 1921 as

> an epidemic syndrome characterized in most instances by a gradual onset with headache, vertigo, disturbances of vision, ocular palsies [inability of individuals to move their eyes normally], changes in speech, dysphagia [difficulty swallowing], marked asthenia [weakness], fever (usually of a low grade), obstinate constipation, incontinence of urine [loss of bladder control], a peculiar mask-like expression of the face, and a state of lethargy which gradually develops in the majority of the recognized cases into a coma that is more or less profound.[2]

But that is, perhaps, too unemotional a definition, and one that jams too many symptoms into a single sentence, to make the horrors of the disease seem real.

Let's begin in 1917 when a young scientist named Constantin von Economo was working at the Wagner-Jauregg clinic in Vienna. He was in the air force during World War I and became the first person in Vienna to be granted an international aviation license. He loved flying hot-air balloons and airplanes. The fact that someone hot-air ballooned as their hobby is already supercool, but von Economo also loved the study of science; he obtained a degree in engineering as well as one in medicine. He was also well read, particularly enjoying works like Goethe's *Faust* and Homer's *Odyssey*. He was a man who was passionately *interested* in the world and the way it worked. Oh, he was also a baron and married to the daughter of a Greek prince. It's baffling that there isn't some sort of historical *Fifty Shades of Grey* based on this guy. When he decided to turn his attention away from flying to psychiatry in 1917, his wife worried he might miss aviation. He replied, "No, there is no longer so much new to do there."[3]

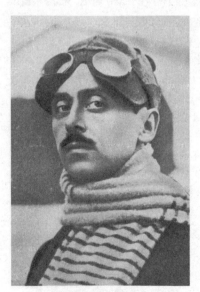

He poses like an advertisement for "adventure."

Fortunately, there was a great deal to study about mental conditions during this period; in that same year Freud wrote his *Introductory Lectures on Psycho-Analysis*. It is kind of odd that the study of certain conditions is considered "fashionable" in some time periods, but if ever studying mental issues was trendy, this was the time and Vienna was the place.

Von Economo soon encountered a wave of patients at the Wagner-Jauregg clinic who all seemed to be suffering from similar symptoms. They came in because their husbands, wives, or children were concerned that they had begun falling asleep inappropriately, for instance, at the dinner table as they were chewing their food or during consultations with their doctor. Patients who fell asleep in front of von Economo would be able to be roused from their stupor, would squint at him briefly, and then go back to sleep.[4]

If you are tempted to exclaim, "That sounds like me on a Monday morning! I hate Mondays!" then:

1. I assume you are Jim Davis. Congratulations on *Garfield*'s success.
2. No, it does not sound like you. You can chew your food without physically collapsing.

There were other symptoms that affected patients in various ways. None resembled needing a nap from time to time. One patient couldn't swallow and regurgitated food through her nostrils. Another couldn't look to the left. Others couldn't control their facial movements. One hallucinated that a group of people surrounded him. Some suffered from "forced laughter."[5] All seemed to be very, very tired, which led von Economo to conclude, "We are dealing with a sleeping sickness."[6]

I would never disparage von Economo, but I'm not sure anyone needed all of the Goethe and Homer and the numerous degrees to figure that out.

When faced with the need for more specifics, von Economo consulted his mother. She told him about a sleeping sickness that had struck parts of Europe in the 1890s that was known as "Nona" or "the living dead." In 1929 von Economo would claim, "Today, we can with some certainty maintain that Nona and Encephalitis Lethargica are identical diseases."[7]

Describing sufferers as "the living dead" is extremely alarming and unfortunately seems like an accurate characterization of the patients von Economo was seeing.

EL didn't necessarily end in death. Only four of von Economo's initial eleven case studies died. Admittedly, that is not a great ratio.[8] But after weeks or months many patients seemed to recover. No doubt von Economo and the doctors treating them, and certainly their families, rejoiced!

They rejoiced too soon.

Though the recovered patients might have seemed "normal" for a prolonged period, even years, few recovered permanently or became their old selves again. Children who had suffered from EL often emerged with altered—for the worse—personalities. Reports surfaced of children who had always been docile turning into truly terrifying adults years after they had "recovered" from the disease. Some children who had been gentle before EL smeared feces on the walls. Some tried to murder their siblings. Some tried to rape and mutilate other children. One tried to bite off another child's penis. In 1928, in one famous case, a sufferer pulled out all her teeth and plucked out her eyes. One doctor claimed, "When the child's personality changes so dramatically, they've 'lost' the original child forever."[9] Even more tragically, unlike psychopaths, the children were largely horrified by their impulses. They even asked to be put away for their own and others' safety, and begged doctors to try to understand how little control they had over their impulses. The lucky ones ended up in asylums. The unlucky ones died or ended their lives in prison.[10]

The aftereffects of EL seemed to manifest differently in adults. The most common chronic effect among adults was the development of Postencephalitic Parkinson's disease. After seeming to recover, many patients then lapsed into an unresponsive state and remained that way for years, prompting von Economo to refer to them as "extinct volcanoes."[11] One patient described the state: "I ceased to have any moods. I ceased to care about anything. Nothing moved me—not even the death of my parents. I forgot what it felt like to be happy or unhappy. Was it good or bad? It was neither. It was nothing."[12] Immobile, unresponsive, and unable to fend for themselves, many would be confined to institutions, where they would need constant care for decades.[13]

If von Economo's theories about Nona are to be believed, there had likely been outbreaks of something similar to EL before. But no one recorded the condition in such scientific terms before the twentieth century. Molly Caldwell Crosby, the author of *Asleep: The Forgotten Epidemic That Remains One of Medicine's Greatest Mysteries*, notes that numerous folktales point to incidences of a disease that closely resembles the one von Economo encountered. You can probably name a lot of them yourself. Let's play a game where we can see how many folktales involving sleeping we can rattle off in under a minute:

1. Sleeping Beauty
2. Snow White
3. Rip Van Winkle

Okay, that is three. Good for us! Are there more? You bet.

Physicians also reported people falling into catatonic stupors with surprising regularity in mid-nineteenth-century Germany. Those reports inspired two of Edgar Allan Poe's most famous stories, "The Fall of the House of Usher" and "The Premature Burial."[14]

Von Economo's new scientific methods—he had a

microscope!—allowed him to pinpoint the physical cause of the disease more accurately than ever before. In his initial paper on the disease, he ruled out toxins caused by food poisoning or malnutrition by determining that his patients had no gastro-intestinal disturbances. He researched his patients' histories to make sure they hadn't been exposed to poisons (for example, poison gas complications experienced by soldiers). He drew spinal fluid to ensure they were not suffering from influenza. They tested negative for syphilis. There was no polio epidemic in Vienna at the time, so it seemed unlikely they had polio. Von Economo did, however, find spherical bacteria formations when he took samples from his deceased patients of the membrane that encased the brain. Those samples would prove especially important as he would later go on to demonstrate that the disease could be transmitted to a monkey through insertion of that bacteria into its brain tissue.[15]

And—this is especially interesting—due to the location of the patients' brain damage, von Economo theorized that the affected brain region, the hypothalamus, regulates sleep. He would be proved correct on that supposition, although not for another seventy years.[16]

Von Economo published his paper on April 27, 1917. Timing being everything, another scientist named Jean-René Cruchet had published a paper on the condition a few days prior. In it he described soldiers he had treated who seemed to be suffering from a disease similar to EL. He *was not happy* about von Economo getting credit for any research on the disease and suggested that, instead of calling it encephalitis lethargica, the world should call it "the disease of Cruchet." Von Economo countered that maybe *one* of Cruchet's forty patients actually had EL; the rest were probably simply suffering from wartime maladies.[17] For a time, in Vienna the disease was known as von Economo's encephalitis lethargica and in France as Cruchet's disease. I am not paying much attention to Cruchet because he did not race balloons. If you want to call EL Cruchet's disease, you can.

Overseas people really weren't calling it much of anything.

If you have never heard of EL—and are marveling that you never knew of a disease that turns people into comatose "living dead" versions of their former selves or children of the damned—well, a lot of people didn't know about it even as the outbreak was happening. Not because the death toll of EL wasn't significant. It was. But it was overshadowed by World War I. (The war overshadowed everything during those years.) And if people weren't paying attention to the war, they were focused on the epidemic of the Spanish flu, which was occurring at the same time. And, as we know, the death toll from that was shockingly high.

Now, you might think to yourself, *Those two diseases occurred at the same time—maybe they were related. Could EL be a symptom of influenza?* You are smart! I, too, considered that possibility, but it didn't exactly pan out. While there is still dispute as to whether the two are connected, von Economo at least strongly felt they weren't. His patients tested negative for influenza. The first case of EL was studied in 1916, before the first reported case of the 1918 influenza epidemic. Moreover, von Economo noted that the high fevers, muscle pain, and upper respiratory symptoms (coughing or sneezing) that accompanied influenza were absent in the presentation of EL.[18] If you are interested in following a line of thought on interrelated diseases, though, some scientists today think that EL is related to streptococcal bacteria, so that's a fun thing to consider when you get strep throat.

In 1918 the first cases of EL appeared in London, baffling clinicians there, who had minimal awareness of the outbreak in Vienna. Professor A. J. Hall wrote:

> They could not find amongst the diseases of their acquaintance a foot which would go into this newly found glass

slipper. A search was therefore made amongst the diseases which, so to say, did not move in Court circles, and were not personally known to the seekers. Amongst those it was at first thought that the owner of the slipper had been found, and that her name was Botulism. After many painstaking efforts to force her foot into the slipper, it was found to be impossible, and the attempt was abandoned. Botulism was not Cinderella.[19]

No, of course it wasn't, because it was EL. Physicians, who initially declared that they were dealing with a wholly new disease,[20] came to their senses and recognized: "For identification and description, it was decided to follow von Economo in terming the illness encephalitis lethargica, a name which has the right of priority and indicates a characteristic clinical feature."[21]

Admittedly, some of the symptoms that sufferers were displaying in London were different from those that had first been observed in Vienna. For instance, the London incarnation of the disease sometimes manifested with bouts of hyperkinetic energy. One boy jumped up and down on all fours, obviously terrified and not in control of his actions at all. Others talked incessantly. But most presented with the same lethargy and sleepiness that had been observed by von Economo in Vienna. And in a super-creepy detail, a lot of the patients slept with their eyes open, which isn't necessarily scarier than someone jumping uncontrollably but really adds to the whole "we're in a horror movie" feel.

In 1918 there were 538 cases of EL in England. The death rate crept up to 50 percent—mostly from paralysis of the respiratory system.[22] And, even more terrifying, it had by now become very clear that among those patients who survived, most weren't going to return to their normal selves. They would live out their lives in institutions.

The disease kept spreading. It made its way to China, India, Australia, Sweden, Uruguay—*all the places*. In New York a neurologist met with a teenage girl's family. She had been sleeping for two months and could respond only insofar as she could blink when told to or squeeze a hand on command. He regretfully told her family that nothing could be done. As he told them, the girl began to cry.

There were some happier cases. In 1920 a woman with EL remained asleep for over three months. Her husband, aware of her great love of music, then hired a musician to play Schubert by her bedside. She woke up immediately and went on to make a full recovery. The *London Times* claimed, "This is the first case in the records of the New York Health Department of a cure in a case of Encephalitis Lethargica."[23] That may have been, and it's a great story, but playing Schubert was not an especially successful cure with anyone else.

Trials for a vaccine began. The Matheson Commission for the Study of Epidemic Encephalitis was founded in 1927, endowed by the industrialist William J. Matheson, who suffered from EL. Josephine B. Neal, who led the research, wrote four influential papers on the disease and became the world's leading expert on EL—but the group had no success in finding a vaccine or a cure. Neal noted "how difficult it was to prove the efficacy of a treatment for EL because of EL's course of natural remissions and progressions."[24] Though Neal continued to work on EL until her death in 1955, in 1942 she sadly wrote to all her patients that the commission had been shut down due to lack of funding.[25]

Twenty-six years after the initial cases of the disease, A. J. Hall's lament—"It may be that generations which follow us will see clearly where we can only grope darkly"—still seemed applicable.[26] This poignant sentiment must resonate with medical researchers throughout every age.

But . . . Remember that cool graph at the beginning of this chapter? Medicine changed really fast!

Stories like the one about the influenza epidemic of 1918 are terrifying because we have become complacently accustomed to thinking that most diseases that killed people in the past are now treatable. That's not the case with influenza! And that's not even the case with EL. However, luckily for the sufferers of EL, medicine progressed so quickly in the twentieth century that its advances offered some relief during their lifetimes.

If that does not immediately take your breath away, consider that a cure for syphilis only came about after people had been having noses grafted onto their syphilitic faces for five hundred years. In the twentieth century (and even now), a disease could be identified, dismissed as tragically untreatable and best left to future generations, and then fifty years later scientific advances would allow for radically, dramatically different treatments. At the beginning of the EL outbreak, it was a really big deal that von Economo had a microscope. In the following years the pace of developments in chemistry and medicine would be breathtaking.

The story of EL is intertwined with the work of Oliver Sacks. Sacks was the coolest man ever to walk the earth. Sorry, Constantin von Economo, I have a fickle heart.

Oliver Sacks was a neurologist and a wonderful author of medical narratives like *The Man Who Mistook His Wife for a Hat*. If you haven't read it, do! You are reading this book, so you presumably like tales about strange medical conditions. All of his writing makes Sacks out to be a compassionate, smart, funny man, which is a view supported by his colleagues and patients and all who knew him.

In his nonfiction account *Awakenings*, Sacks discusses how he "awakened" some of the longtime sufferers of EL. I will let him set the scene because I have nothing on him in the "writing nonfiction about medicine" game. Sacks explains in the foreword to *Awakenings* that early in 1969

these "extinct volcanoes" erupted into life. The placid atmosphere of Mount Carmel was transformed—occurring before us was a cataclysm of almost geological proportions, the explosive "awakening," the "quickening," of eighty or more patients who had long been regarded, and regarded themselves, as effectively dead.[27]

Sacks recalled it as "the most significant and extraordinary event in my life." Yes, Oliver Sacks basically brought people back from the dead! Someone get out the confetti! Pop the champagne because we are bringing Lazarus back and you *know* that guy loves bubbly!

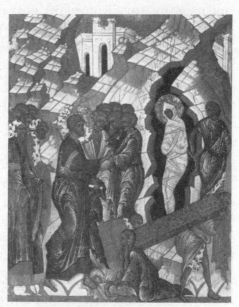

Lazarus is wearing a cozy outfit and he is ready to par-TAY.

Sacks's patients' miraculous awakenings seem especially unlikely when you consider the fact that by the 1960s, EL wasn't even covered in medical school. This would have made von Economo really angry, as he once noted: "One thing is certain: whoever has observed without bias the many forms of encephalitis lethargica . . . must of necessity have quite considerably altered his outlook on neurological and psychological phenomena . . . Encephalitis lethargica can scarcely again be forgotten."[28] Wrong, Constantin. People often take whatever information about the world makes them feel scared or dumb and stuff it away as quickly as possible.

It must therefore have been something of a surprise to Sacks to begin his appointment at Beth Abraham Home for the Incurables (renamed Mount Carmel in his book) and find eighty post-encephalitic patients. He noted: "Almost half of these patients were immersed in states of pathological 'sleep,' virtually speechless and motionless, and requiring total nursing-care; the remainder were less disabled, less dependent, less isolated, and less depressed, could look after many of their own basic needs, and maintain a modicum of personal and social life."[29]

Sacks first attempted to give these patients a basic sense of self by trying to find their lost relatives and then persuading those people to visit. He also formed close relationships with them himself. He found that some of the patients were more responsive than initially considered. However, they were only reactive if stimulus seemed to come from the outside world.[30]

As depicted in the movie *Awakenings* (1990), if you threw patients a ball, they could catch it. That wasn't just the case with patients at Beth Abraham; a patient in the Highlands Hospital in London, if thrown a ball, would play with it so energetically that the staff nicknamed him Puskás (after the great Hungarian soccer player). Other patients could walk if you supported them. Unfortunately, they had no will to do so on their own. Sadly, basic responses to the outside world are not nearly enough to constitute a full life. There is a big difference between being able to catch a ball when someone tosses it at you and being able to say, "I would like to play with a ball now" and then get one.[31]

Most of Sacks's fellow doctors had dismissed these patients as chronic cases for which little could be done. The fact that Sacks took the time to understand their symptoms and interact with them at all is great. Let's pause to say, "What a nice guy!" And then L-dopa came along. In 1969 Sacks began testing large doses of a new promising anti-Parkinson drug called Levodopa or, more commonly L-dopa, on the patients at Beth Abraham.

The results were extraordinary. Patients who had been barely responsive for years remarkably returned to their old personalities, admittedly in much older bodies. A man who had raced cars until the 1930s awoke and, although he could no longer take to the road, began drawing highly realistic cars. Sacks reported: "His cars were accurate, authentic, and had an odd charm. When he was not drawing, he was talking, or writing—of 'the old days' in the twenties when he was driving and racing."[32] One woman woke and, though she could inform the doctors of the dates of momentous occasions like Pearl Harbor, believed that she was still age twenty-one and that the year was still 1926. Sacks wrote that she "spoke of Gershwin and other contemporaries as if they were still alive; of events in the mid-twenties as if they had just happened. She had obsolete mannerisms and turns of speech; she gave the impression of a 'flapper' come suddenly to life." She could, understandably, not imagine what it was like to be older than 21 because she had never done any of the things that we associate with aging.[33]

Sacks later recalled: "What I . . . regret, and what many of the patients did as well, was that this [L-dopa] was not available 10 or 20 years before, when they had not lost so many of their connections to the world."[34] He claimed that the twenty-one-year-old flapper was one of the patients whom he found the saddest, but I think that party-girl flappers are resilient and generally happy to be alive.

No *wonder* this phenomenon was made into a movie! How terrible to awake feeling you had thirty or forty years of your life ripped away from you. But how amazing to see these people suddenly return to their full selves.

There were downsides. The patients suffered from physical side effects—like respiratory attacks—as well as the psychological difficulties that stemmed from having lost so many years. But they had their minds and their energy, their quirks and passions and interests. After so many years of shadowy half-life, how wonderful it must have been for them to return to the world.

But, tragically, the effects of L-dopa didn't last. Many of the patients were overwhelmed by tics. Some exhibited manic behavior. Sacks recalled one patient who "liked exchanging kisses with the nurses. Then the erotic fantasies became more extreme. He wanted a brothel service to be set up."[35] This is very unfortunate, but I have seen the movie *One Flew Over the Cuckoo's Nest* (1975) enough times to appreciate that guy's style. The experiment was discontinued, although some of Sacks's patients continued to receive L-dopa until the end of their lives. The drug is still used to treat Parkinson's today, but many patients experience a "wearing off" effect after four to six years.[36]

Sacks's patients fell back into their former states and could not be awakened again. Does that mean that their brief awakening was meaningless? Well, if life is only important if it is going to last forever, the whole human race is in bad shape. One patient, who before L-dopa had been so hunched that she was forced to always stare at the ground, went on a day trip to a local park while experiencing her awakening. When she came back she said, "What a perfect day—so peaceful—I shall never forget it! It's a joy to be alive on a day like this. And I do feel alive, more truly alive than I've felt in twenty years. If this is what L-DOPA can do, it's an absolute blessing!"[37] Another patient claimed, following his awakening, "If people felt as good as I did, nobody would make wars."[38]

At the end of our lives I think many of us would do anything to have one more good day. All of this life seems so precious. I can't think of anything as a failure that allows people even one more happy day. Sacks claimed: "They were not only patients but teachers and friends, the years I spent with them were the most significant of my life. I want something of their lives, their presence, to be preserved and live for others, as exemplars of human predicament and survival."[39]

There is still no cure for EL, and its rise and subsequent disappearance is still regarded as something of a mystery. But if within a time span of fifty years we can research a disease and come up with a drug that can bring people back, even if only temporarily, imagine what we will be able to do in the next fifty. The sufferers of this disease won't be the only ones awakened. If we study and research and devote energies to science, hopefully there will be many Lazarus bodies dancing to and fro through the parks in our lifetime.

Lobotomies

*I'd rather have a free bottle in
front of me than a prefontal
lobotomy.*

—Tom Waits

As we learned from my excellent line drawing in the last chapter, medical science advanced at an astonishing pace in the twentieth century. On the whole, that is wonderful. That is a great boon for humanity. But there can be a downside to new medical science, as when it is wielded by a charismatic demagogue who cares more about his own reputation than the well-being of his patients.

Now, there have always been charlatans who claimed to have cures for dangerous diseases despite having no such thing (see: Alexander of Abonoteichos of the useless charms for the Antonine plague). Their outrageous conduct meant that patients often died—a good indication that their treatment didn't work. However, with scientific advances, quacks could offer more than just charms to ward off disease. By the twentieth century medical science had advanced to a point where unscrupulous individuals could cause irreversible damage to patients without actually killing them. And then they could call their procedures "successes." And people were not vigilant enough, or not sufficiently aware, to say, "No, that is not what success means." What happens when a "cure" causes more harm than good?

Which brings us to lobotomies, the scariest procedure that you never want performed. This is a plague induced by human stupidity, not disease, but I couldn't write a book on deadly medical horrors without talking about the terror wreaked by Walter Jackson Freeman II.

The first leucotomy or lobotomy was performed on a human by the Portuguese neurologist Antônio Egas Moniz in 1935. This operation involved drilling holes into a patient's skull and then making cuts into the brain's frontal lobes to sever their connections to the rest of the brain.[1]

He was inspired by a similar surgery that had been performed on chimpanzees at Yale University. According to "The Lobotomist," an episode in the PBS TV series (2010) *American Experience*, "Two chimps, Becky and Lucy . . . showed that once their frontal lobes were removed, they lost the capacity to solve simple problems." But scientists also noticed that Becky was no longer frustrated when she was unable to solve problems. She was not bothered in the way a puzzle-solving chimpanzee should be at all. Dr. Carlyle Jacobsen, who performed the procedure, claimed that she seemed to have joined a "happiness cult" or "placed her burdens on the Lord."[2] Lucy didn't seem so happy, but absolutely no one paid attention to her. You could say that they . . . *did not love Lucy*. (That joke would have gone over gangbusters in 1950.)

There was some precedence for these observations—and with a human, not a mellow chimpanzee. In the 1840s there was a well-known medical case involving a man named Phineas Gage who had survived having an iron bar driven into his frontal lobes. While he recovered physically, his personality was so severely altered that he seemed to be "a child in his intellectual capacity and manifestations."[3] By 1871 the Scottish neurologist David Ferrier had separately discovered that intellect seemed to reside in the frontal lobes of the brain.

The takeaway from the chimp experiment should have been, "Well, that was interesting. But let's not mess around with anyone's frontal lobes. Let's just not do that. This whole experiment was just a reminder about intellect and problem solving. Okay, we are all agreed. Let's have lunch." But Becky's response to the procedure stood out. A reduction in anxiety and negative emotion is striking and, at first glance, seems like a very good result.

Dr. Moniz believed that such an operation would make life far better for the insane. And if "better life" just constitutes "being less worried and agitated," he was correct. There is one problem, though: worrying about stuff serves a purpose. It's not fun and can keep you awake at night, but it means you are capable of caring and solving problems. Which means you are qualified to be an empathetic, adult human being.

Dr. Moniz was not considering the disadvantages of a life without worry.

The first lobotomies involved drilling two holes about three centimeters deep directly into a patient's skull over the frontal lobes. Then alcohol was injected into the frontal lobes in an attempt to disrupt neural pathways. When the ethyl alcohol proved less than entirely effective, Moniz and his team began cutting the lobe with wire, using an instrument called the leucotome. A wire loop extended from the end of a handle and would be rotated in a circle to cut neural fibers. They didn't actually remove the frontal lobes, à la a casual dinner party with Hannibal Lecter; they just severed the connections between the frontal lobes and the rest of the brain. That's a delicate bit of neurosurgery but only took around an hour to complete.

Unlike Moniz, Walter Jackson Freeman II, while a physician, was not a surgeon, let alone a neurosurgeon. This man had no business whatsoever operating on any part of the body, but he *especially* should not have been operating on an organ as delicate as the brain. That did not stop him. He and his partner James Watts performed the first version of this surgery in the United States in 1936. Their patient was a sixty-three-year-old woman named Alice Hammatt. She suffered from severe depression—perhaps aggravated by the fact that one of her children had died, as had her sister and brother-in-law in a murder-suicide pact. She entertained thoughts of suicide. Moreover, according to Freeman, she was just no fun to be around. She was "a master at bitching and really led her husband a dog's life . . . She worried if he was a few minutes late in coming from the office and raised the roof when things did not suit her."[4] No one seemingly pointed out that severe depression is a valid and understandable response to the tremendous amount of unexpected death that had touched Ms. Hammatt. Also, it's nice when people are punctual. People should text if they're going to be late; it's just respectful.

After the operation Hammatt was free from anxiety. That said, after the operation she was also only able to flip through magazines and draw pictures. She misspelled words on her pictures when she tried to caption them. She wasn't able to have a coherent conversation. She ultimately regained her ability to speak, although "her husband and maid did most of the work" around her home, according to Freeman. But she was very happy with the procedure and felt that she spent a lot less time worrying. She was even able to spend pleasant time with acquaintances she had before found extremely annoying. Freeman thought "the result was spectacular."

This may just be me, but the thought of finding the people I consider annoying suddenly agreeable strikes me as anything but a spectacular result.

Perhaps the most famous example of a lobotomy gone very wrong was Rosemary Kennedy, the daughter of Rose and

Joseph P. Kennedy and one of the sisters of President John F. Kennedy. The third Kennedy child, Rosemary was always a little bit slower than the rest of her extremely competitive siblings. But, to be fair, all of us are a little slower than the ultracompetitive, hyperathletic, superattractive *Übermench*es that are the Kennedy clan.

Rosemary was born in Boston in September 1918. *I think we all know what was happening then.* Or, in case you like reading chapters out of order—I do!—the influenza epidemic was devastating the United States. A doctor was supposed to come to the Kennedy household when Rosemary's mother went into labor, but he was delayed because he was treating so many influenza patients. The nurse at the Kennedy home told Rosemary's mother to cross her legs and try to hold on until the doctor got there, which she did. When Rosemary still appeared to be coming, the nurse *pushed the baby back into the birth canal.*

The shortage of oxygen during her birth resulting from this clear case of medical malpractice likely caused brain damage; Rosemary's IQ was later estimated to be low. How low precisely isn't known, though she attended a school that accepted girls with IQs of 65 to 90. Did this mean she had an unhappy life? No, of course not! Forrest Gump's IQ was 75, and he had a *great* life. He played Ping-Pong and traveled the world and everything! Rosemary was hardworking, affectionate, and fiercely devoted to her family. She was also very good with children. Those all seem like qualities that contribute to a pleasant and fulfilling existence. As she grew older, however, and her other siblings moved on to their own seemingly more exciting lives, Rosemary became increasingly prone to temper tantrums. Her father, Joseph, was terrified that she'd have premarital sex, possibly get pregnant, and embarrass the family at a time when he was mapping out his sons' political careers. In 1941, when Rosemary was age twenty-three, he decided a lobotomy might be a cure for her unpredictable behavior. Spoiler for all of history: Joseph Kennedy was a monster.

Rosemary's sister Kathleen (known as Kick) investigated the procedure and was told by a reporter who was writing a series on the treatment that lobotomized people "don't worry so much, but they're gone as a person, just gone."[5] *Journal of the American Medical Association* wrote: "It is inconceivable that a procedure which effectively destroys the function of this portion of the brain could possibly restore the person concerned to a wholly normal state."[6]

None of this information deterred Joseph Kennedy. He engaged Freeman and Watts to perform a lobotomy on Rosemary. She was kept awake for the procedure as they asked her to recite the lyrics to simple songs like "God Bless America" and the months of the year. They kept cutting until she became incoherent.[7] After the operation she was unable to walk or talk. She was incontinent. Some of her siblings stopped visiting her. Even with years of rehabilitative efforts, she was only ever able to speak a few words. The nurse who assisted at the operation quit the profession altogether.[8]

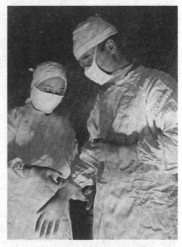

However, at the time the public never learned about what happened to Rosemary or cases like hers. It was in neither the Kennedy family's nor Freeman and Watts's interest to let people know about the horrifying effects of her operation.

Results like these weren't enough to deter Freeman. Remarkably, he came to think that Moniz's technique was not efficient enough to lobotomize

What's so scary about this?

all the people who he believed could benefit from the procedure. He and his partner thought that the drilling was the most bothersome part for patients. They claimed: "Apprehension becomes a little more marked when the holes are drilled, probably because of the actual pressure on the skull and the grinding sound that is as distressing, or more so, than the drilling of a tooth."[9] I would go with "more so."

So they developed the transorbital lobotomy, which involved inserting an ice pick into a patient's skull through the bone known as the orbit at the back of the eye socket. Patients were generally subdued with electroshock therapy beforehand. Then the ice pick was driven through the back of the eye with a hammer. There, it would be moved back and forth in the same motion as an eggbeater, severing connections between the thalamus (which controls the motor systems of the brain, extending to basic functions like movement and consciousness) and frontal lobes (which regulate higher intellect). The operation itself could be performed in less than ten minutes, and as soon as the bleeding stopped, patients were sent home (generally in a taxi) just as if they had been to the dentist.[10]

Freeman certainly wanted to make this procedure seem like it was no big deal. Which is outrageous. Bear in mind that after a lobotomy a lot of the patients could barely remember who they were when they were being herded into a taxi. If they read something, they couldn't recall it afterward. Many fumbled with their genitals. Despite Freeman and Watts's frequent comparisons to going to the dentist, I beg to differ. Going to the dentist sucks, but afterward you can remember who you are: namely, a person with a sore mouth who wishes you had not just been to the dentist.

In 1946 Freeman performed his new transorbital operation on Sallie Ellen Ionesco. She was severely depressed, so much so that she stayed in bed for days at a time. She had tried to com-mit suicide, and she had tried to smother one of her children. It does indeed seem like her quality of life was not great. After the lobotomy she was never violent again. When she was interviewed about it later, she claimed, "[Freeman] was a great man, that's all I can say . . . I don't remember nothing else, and I'm very tired." Her daughter, however, did say that she wished Freeman "hadn't gotten quite so out of hand."[11]

Many of the people who were lobotomized were untroubled by the results. According to John B. Dynes and James L. Poppen in their 1949 *American Medical Journal* article "Lobotomy for Intractable Pain," after patients were operated on, "they never admitted they were mentally depressed and at no time did they show grief or shed tears."[12] However, all of the patients that Dynes and Poppen surveyed who before their lobotomies had been classified as "normal" or in some cases in an "anxiety state" were afterward classified as "retarded" or "euphoric" (which, as far as I can tell, meant "mentally impaired but pleased about it"). In addition to feeling no depression: "They were indifferent to sorrow or grief, and seemed incapable of sensing or appreciating the feelings of others."[13]

Often Freeman was inclined to see his operations as successful, while those closer to the patients saw them as anything but. Regarding the "success" of the operation on a twenty-four-year-old schizophrenic, Freeman reported: "Except for drinking too much, he presents no aggressive misbehavior. It apparently requires some imagination, as well as some emotional driving force, to bring about misbehavior at the legally reprehensible level and this the patient is incapable of."[14] Okay, that's sort of nice that the patient wasn't doing anything illegal. However, that patient probably did not have time to misbehave given his brother's statement that "he had lost all sense of time, spending four to six hours a day washing his hands but nevertheless going around with dirty clothes."[15]

The more lobotomies Freeman performed, the more obvious the disadvantages of the operation became. Even Freeman admitted, "Every patient probably loses something by this operation, some spontaneity, some sparkle, some flavor of the personality."[16]

What is that elusive "sparkle"? Is it a certain panache that accompanies the telling of one's stories? An almost Fitzgeraldian gleam in someone's eye as they exclaim, "To the wine cellar, Maurice! We're going to fill this bathtub with champagne!"

Nope. That "sparkle" was "adult intellect."

Discover magazine lays out the situation more clearly: "The operation did have disturbing side effects. Patients often suffered major personality changes and became apathetic, prone to inappropriate social behavior, and infatuated with their own toilet habits. They told pointless jokes and exhibited poor hygiene."[17] So they often behaved like toddlers. The granddaughter of a woman who was operated on in 1953 claimed that afterward "she was strange because she would do things like rock in place. She didn't make a lot of sense when she talked. And she didn't talk about the same things that other adults talked about. She was— childlike is probably the best description."[18]

Freeman didn't seem to regard a reversion to toddler-hood as a distressing outcome. Of a patient he operated on in 1947 in an attempt to treat her schizophrenia, he reported:

[Postoperative day 10] Rose is a smiling, lazy and satisfactory patient with the personality of an oyster. She pours and pours from an empty coffee pot. She can't remember my name.

[Postoperative day 18] Rose is delighted to be going home. She doesn't say much, is very ticklish.[19]

Rose was a married woman in her late twenties. When relatives responded with horror at her condition, Freeman suggested that if she misbehaved she might be in need of "a good old fashioned spanking . . . followed by a dish of icecream [*sic*], then a kiss and make up."[20]

If people had been vibrant creators prior to their lobotomies, well, that creativity was gone afterward. Dyne and Poppen explained:

> As an example, one patient was an inventor, and although after lobotomy he was euphoric and restless and showed no distinct intellectual or memory deficit, he was totally incapable of creative work or the visualization of a problem. He was unable to concentrate or to plan for the future. He seemed to lack interest or actually to be able to maintain an interest for more than a few minutes at a time.[21]

It seemed the best possible outcome of a lobotomy was the patient's retention of at least *some* personality. Freeman's son later scoffed, "You could never talk about a successful lobotomy. You might as well talk about a successful automobile accident."[22]

In 1949 Freeman took to the road to demonstrate his procedure at hospitals across the country. He traveled in a custom-fitted Lincoln Continental he dubbed the lobotomobile—like an ice cream truck manned by a demon. In the vehicle Freeman carried with him a portable electroshock machine, a tape recorder for his notes, and his instruments. He toured eight states over five weeks and performed 111 operations.[23]

Freeman was a consummate showman. His partner James Watts described him as "a barker at a carnival." He had a theatrical disposition that might even have been evidenced by his attire. At one point Freeman had cut a ring off a man's penis, which he engraved with his family crest and wore around his neck for years afterward. In the course of demonstrating his lobotomy procedure, he would sometimes wield carpenter's mallets in both hands so as to drive icepicks into both eye sockets simultaneously. One person who observed him at work recalled: "He looked up at us, smiling. I thought I was seeing a circus act. He moved both hands back and forth in unison, cutting the brain identically behind each eye. It astonished me that he was so gay, so high, so 'up.'"[24]

If you are thinking, *Whoa, that is not the measured behavior I expect from a doctor!* you are right. This was a nightmare carnival. Someone who was traveling from place to place doing dozens of these operations week after week was probably not taking this surgery as seriously as . . . basically any medical procedure deserves.

According to one of Freeman's assistants, a patient got cold feet and decided not to go ahead with a lobotomy. Freeman went to his hotel, presumably to reason with him, and brought along his electroshock machine, planning to administer a few volts to calm him. The patient began running away, screaming, *from a man who had shown up at his hotel room to lobotomize him.* That reaction seems extremely sane. Freeman was not deterred. The assistant claimed, "The patient was . . . held down on the floor while Freeman administered the shock. It then occurred to him that since the patient was already unconscious, and he had a set of leucotomes in his pocket, he might as well do the transorbital lobotomy then and there, which he did."[25] He cut into an unwilling man's brain in an unsterilized hotel room. After wrestling him to the ground.

Freeman didn't worry about what he referred to as "all that germ crap."[26] I tried to think of a medical procedure that could reasonably be treated so cavalierly, and honestly, I think I'd show more bedside manner bandaging a child's scraped knee.

In spite of these downsides, which, again, seem utterly horrific, *people lined up for lobotomies*, especially since it was possible to get it done without skull drilling and instead with that nifty ice pick. For some perspective on how many of these operations Freeman was performing, you can look at some of his notes as he traveled across the country:

29 June, Little Rock, Arkansas, 4 patients
30 June, Rusk, Texas, 10 patients
1 July, Terrell, Texas, 7 patients
2 July, Wichita Falls, Texas, 3 patients
9 July, Patton, California, 5 patients
14 July, Berkeley, California, 3 patients[27]

That's thirty-two lobotomies in about two weeks. Two lobotomies a day.

Now, why would so many people want a lobotomy?

The popularity of the procedure was due to the fact that, at the time, there were very limited treatments available to help the mentally ill. "When I visited mental hospitals," recalled the retired neurosurgeon Jason Brice, attempting to explain the popularity of the lobotomy during these years, "you saw straitjackets, padded cells, and it was patently apparent that some of the patients were, I'm sorry to say, subjected to physical violence."[28] Asylums, prior to the rise of medications that could help or at least subdue patients, often acted as little more than holding pens where ill and sometimes violent people were kept. Treatments at the time included electroshock therapy—which is still used to treat some severe cases of depression today—but it could result in memory loss. The drug Metrazol induced convulsions so intense that patients broke their bones, in some cases their spines and jaws. Insulin comas kept patients unconscious for weeks. These treatments offered a bit of relief in some cases, but not at the rate doctors might have hoped.

The physicians performing lobotomies were so desperate for a cure that they were easily susceptible to false hope. In desperate times, who isn't? Suddenly, there seemed to be a procedure that offered patients at least the possibility of relief. There was a fix that was supposed to be permanent and quick and easy to perform. No harder than a dental procedure, really!

In the late 1940s many Americans were suffering from

mental afflictions. World War II had ended, and soldiers were having difficulties readjusting to civilian life. Many were suffering from post-traumatic stress disorder (PTSD)—many still do—probably because *they had been to war*. There was no medical term for their condition yet, but Veterans Affairs (VA) hospitals were bursting at the seams. A 1955 National Research Council study claimed that during World War II 1.2 million soldiers had been admitted for psychiatric and neurological problems.[29] For comparison, 680,000 were admitted for physical injuries from battle. One treatment, among others popular at the time, consisted of spraying the soldiers with alternating hot and cold water under extremely high pressure. It was nicknamed a "Scotch Douche and Needle Shower."[30] There's no time when being thrown unexpectedly into water of an uncomfortable temperature has really calmed anyone down or cheered anyone up, which gives the strong impression that people were just trying things at random and hoping one would work.

This was the twentieth century, not the Dark Ages. Einstein and Frank Sinatra were walking around.

In 1946 VA chief Frank Hines received a memo that declared: "Approximately 6 years ago a French surgeon, Egas Moniz, described an operation on the pre-frontal lobes of the brain . . . the operation has been found of value in eliminating apprehension, anxiety, depression and compulsions and obsessions with a marked emotional component . . . Reports of the result are almost uniformly good when the patients are chosen carefully."[31]

Now—and this is the least important problem with the memo—Egas Moniz was Portuguese. He was not French. I know that seems like *such* an easy slipup, especially at a time before Internet searches were commonplace. I'd never normally mention it, but in this case I'm bringing it up because Moniz was the most Portuguese man in the history of Portugal. He was born in Portugal, worked in Portugal, was in the Portuguese parliament, served as an ambassador for Portugal, became Portugal's minister of foreign affairs, attended the Paris Peace Conference in 1919 on behalf of Portugal, was a professor at the largest university in Portugal, and died, also, in Portugal. If he was known for one thing other than inventing the lobotomy, it was being Portuguese.

So I don't think whoever was writing this memo was very familiar with the players in the lobotomy game.

If you are more bothered by the remark that "results were almost uniformly good," you are the kind of person who *can* see the forest for the trees, so good for you.

Frank Hines approved the procedure in the memo despite the fact that much of this note is vague, and wherever it is not vague, it's incorrect. Between April 1, 1947, and September 30, 1950, 1,464 veterans were lobotomized at VA hospitals by VA doctors.[32]

There were other victims of the lobotomy's popularity. Mentally ill women were generally institutionalized by their husbands or fathers—without consent required—and, until the 1960s, doctors were not obliged to reveal their treatments or risks to the patients. "I usually asked the family to provide the patient with sunglasses [for their black eyes postoperation] rather than explanations," Freeman joked.[33] Somewhere between 60 and 80 percent of lobotomies were performed on women, despite a greater percentage of men being institutionalized.[34] Women often went into the surgery thinking the risks were radically less serious than they actually were. For instance, one of Freeman's patients was worried that the operation would mean having her head shaved and losing her beautiful hair. He promised her they would try to avoid cutting off her curls, but they cut her hair anyway. Freeman found her vanity hilarious considering the fact that afterward she would "go about or talk with others quite oblivious to the fact" that she was bald.[35]

What a jokester! As far as I can tell, every single one of

Dr. Freeman's witticisms hinged on how you could rip away someone's higher functioning skills and they would not even know. *Isn't that hilarious?* Sometimes I make jokes about topics that seem scary and dark and people's monocles pop right off—just fly across the room—but American husbands sure did seem to love this man who was driving around in a van chopping up their wives' brains.

The fact that there are situations where it might be advantageous to control an unruly wife or daughter is probably obvious to anyone who has seen *Suddenly, Last Summer.* (Spoiler: to be fair, absolutely no one was ever lobotomized for the very specific cannibalism-related reasons noted in that 1958 Tennessee Williams play.) Some of the women on Dyne and Poppen's list of patients were listed simply as "menopausal" or "hysterical." The historian Kate Clifford Larson wrote: "Freeman would later describe potential patients as society's 'misfits.' Women, in particular, made up the largest group of lobotomy patients. Women who were depressed, had bi-polar illness or were sexually active outside the range of socially and culturally acceptable limits of the day—including single women exhibiting typical sexual desire—were considered candidates."[36] So if you are a standard, twenty-first-century woman who likes reading about diseases rather than . . . well, I am not entirely sure what wholly inoffensive book a woman could read—a cookbook, maybe? One of those books where movie stars tell you to do yoga? Just take it as a given that if you were a married woman who lived during the height of the lobotomy's popularity, your husband would have been able to have you institutionalized and lobotomized if he felt like it. To my married female readers: of course I do not mean *your* husband. I am sure your husband is a really cool guy. But still. He could have.

Unlike your husband, Freeman was deeply uncool. He never ceased to believe that the lobotomy was something of a miracle cure, and continually presented it as such. He was a master at working with the press from the very beginning. As early as 1937 he described the procedure to the *New York Times* in such a way that the paper published an article poetically declaring it "Surgery Used on the Soul Sick." Freeman claimed, "Watts and I had made the headlines even though we did not get an award. He and I worked hard on that one and talked ourselves hoarse."[37] Meanwhile an article in the *Washington Evening Star* after Freeman's sixth operation described the procedure as one that "probably constitutes one of the greatest surgical innovations of this generation."[38] He had an amazing catchphrase—"Get them home!"—in regard to his patients, which certainly preyed on distressed family members' sensibilities.

After these articles appeared, Freeman would hear from many people who wanted lobotomies. He recalled that there "was a man who complained of asthma and wanted to know if a brain operation would relieve that."[39] I worry that people will read this and think, *Ha-ha, that guy sure was dumb in addition to being asthmatic.* First of all, okay, that's possible, but I am inclined to say the fault is with Freeman. If the man who invented lobotomies couldn't explain the procedure well enough to make it clear that it has nothing to do with a lung disease, he was advertising it in a dangerous way. He made lobotomies sound like a cure-all for everything.

To my knowledge, he didn't operate on that man with the asthma. Which is shocking, as Freeman often lobotomized people who wrote to him, claiming in 1946, "If we waited for psychiatrists to send patients to us we'd still be on our first hundred cases instead of our fifth hundred."[40] Seemingly, that wheezy fellow and the actress Frances Farmer were the only people Freeman didn't enthusiastically lobotomize. (Her parents refused to give their consent to the operation. Nevertheless, some people still believe that the movie star might have been lobotomized. She wasn't. We should focus on the people who were. God knows there are enough of them.)

Freeman used lobotomies to treat everything from "excessive eating" to drug addiction to alcoholism. Freeman's fifteenth patient was an alcoholic. The doctor was convinced a lobotomy would stop his cravings. It didn't work. Immediately following the operation the patient escaped and went to a bar, where Freeman later found him extremely intoxicated. In the 1950s Freeman lobotomized a woman suffering from nothing more than severe headaches. According to her daughter, Carol Noelle, the procedure left the patient with the mind of a small child. She described her mother's lobotomized condition:

> Did she worry about stuff? Nope, didn't worry. Just as Freeman promised, she didn't worry. She had no concept of social graces . . . The only outlet she had was beating every pinball machine in town and knowing how many pennies were in the jar at the carnival, you know. She was the greatest playmate we ever had and the best friend, and we loved her to death. But I never remember calling her mama or mommy or anything. I never even thought of my mother as my daughter's grandmother, and I never even took my daughter to see her, not one time. So she never even got to have that.[41]

I imagine if she had known that she would never have a chance to be with her granddaughter, she would have suffered with the headaches. (Especially had she known that acetaminophen [used in Tylenol] and ibuprofen [found in Advil] would be introduced in 1955 and 1974, respectively.)

One bright spot: Freeman's cavalier attitude toward the downsides of the procedure at least enraged his fellow scientists. James Poppen wrote in 1949: "I do hope that in the future we will not be informed initially through the weekly popular magazines. Any procedure which is instituted for such a serious condition should be thoroughly tried and proved to a certain degree before it is advised. Premature information through weekly magazines (not always accurate) has a tendency to give patients or relatives false hopes or impressions."[42] That remark was relatively polite. My favorite story about Freeman-hate involves him going up to the psychiatrist Henry Stack Sullivan at a cocktail party in 1948 and cheerfully remarking, "How goes it, Harry?" Sullivan raised his hands heavenward in a fury and shouted, "Why do you persist in annoying me?" before, still enraged, he was dragged away by his friend.[43] If I had been at that event, Dr. Sullivan and I would have formed a firm and lasting friendship, but that is beside the point.

Dr. Florence Powdermaker, chief of the VA's psychiatric-education section, wrote a reference note in 1948, wondering, "Has Dr. Freeman shown any disposition to modify his idea that lobotomy is useful for practically everything from delinquency to a pain in the neck?"[44] I am delighted that a female doctor would express some hesitation about this particular treatment. Meanwhile the neurologist (and later president of the American Neurological Association) Lewis Pollock declared almost immediately after Freeman's first operation that lobotomies were "not an operation but a mutilation."[45]

By 1950 the Soviet Union banned lobotomies as "contrary to the principles of humanity."[46]

And did everyone in the United States agree? No. Not really. This was an era when we loved everything the Soviets hated and might well have been referring to vodka as "Freedom Whiskey." Moniz had just won the Nobel Prize for pioneering the surgery in 1949. That same year 5,000 lobotomies were performed in the United States.[47] Altogether, approximately 40,000 lobotomies were performed in the United States between the 1930s and 1970s; Freeman would singlehandedly perform 3,500 of them.[48]

The decline of the lobotomy's popularity took just about

as long as its rise. The change in public opinion required a group of people as passionate about discrediting lobotomies as Freeman was about defending them. Fortunately, as early as the 1950s, journalists and artists began portraying lobotomies in a skeptical light. In 1951 the journalist Irving Wallace wrote an article in the *Saturday Evening Post* titled "The Operation of Last Resort." It was originally called "They Cut Away His Conscience," but that title was judged a bit too controversial (although it appears under that name in Wallace's collection, *The Sunday Gentleman*). In the story, the journalist profiled an exceptionally intelligent man. (He had an IQ of 150! He never stopped reading! He went to Princeton! Good stuff all around!) However, that man was also severely depressed. He had a mental breakdown after being discharged from the army and, after trying a number of psychiatric treatments, was lobotomized. He was happier afterward, but, as Wallace reported—and I don't think this is a surprise given the article's title—*they cut away his conscience.* Wallace wrote: "Prefrontal lobotomy converts patients into docile, inert, often useless drones, stripping them of their old powers, giving them convulsive seizures, making them indifferent to social amenities, filling them with aggressive misbehavior and impairing their foresight and insight. There are those who feel the operation tampers with God's substance, who feel that if it cuts out a man's cares, it also cuts out his soul and his conscience."[49]

The work received a deluge of responses from interested and frightened readers. Good. Well done, Irving Wallace. Freeman *hated* this article. He wanted his name left out of it entirely and, in what I think is a hilariously petulant move, wrote Wallace a letter quoting from the poem "If—" by Rudyard Kipling: "If you can bear to hear the truth you've spoken / Twisted by knaves to make a trap for fools . . . Then you'll be a Man, my son!" But he knew full well that patients could be rendered, among other things, conscienceless. In a 1945 letter to a medical colleague about a former patient of his he wrote: "Your description of her brings up a picture of a rather childish individual with many enthusiasms, with petulance and lofty intransigence but no real deep feelings of distress and **certainly no conscience** [emphasis added] . . . it will be well to see her as an over-sized child rather than as a responsible adult."[50]

There would be more artists who wrote about the damaging impact of lobotomies. Tennessee Williams's beloved sister Rose was lobotomized in 1943, and references to the operation appear overtly in *Suddenly, Last Summer* (1958) and more subtly in *The Glass Menagerie* (1944). In *Menagerie*, after the Rose-esque character's favorite ornament, a unicorn, is broken, she smiles and remarks, "I'll just imagine he had an operation. The horn was removed to make him feel less—freakish! Now he will feel more at home with the other horses, the ones that don't have horns." And then, of course, there is Ken Kesey's 1962 book *One Flew Over the Cuckoo's Nest*, which could well be subtitled *Lobotomies Are Bad and So Is Conformity.*

I wish this was a case of "artists can change the world!" They can! They do! Keep doing art! However, while these depictions inspired the horror with which we regard lobotomies today, the major cause of lobotomies' waning popularity was the introduction of Thorazine in 1955. This antipsychotic medication could effectively quiet and subdue some patients (like schizophrenics) without irreversible side effects. It was first marketed as a "chemical lobotomy."

None of this stopped Freeman, though. Throughout the 1960s he continued to operate—sometimes on children as young as age twelve. Howard Dully, who later recounted the experience in *My Lobotomy*, was operated upon in 1960 because his stepmother claimed: "He objects to going to bed but then sleeps well. He does a good deal of daydreaming and when asked about it he says, 'I don't know.' He turns the room's lights on when there is broad sunlight outside."[51] Turning the lights on during daytime is (1) not all that bad a behavior and (2) something that could likely be changed by saying, "Hey, stop turning all the lights on when it's bright outside, kid; you're going to get grounded if you keep killing us with this electricity bill."

Freeman's license was finally revoked in 1967 when a patient in his care died as Freeman performed his *third* lobotomy on her. As late as 1968 he claimed that he thought lobotomies would make a comeback and that surgeons who were disinclined to perform them were "missing a good bet."[52] That same year he began what he called "the great manhunt of 1968." Before his death in 1972 from cancer, Freeman traveled across the country visiting with his former patients. Many were pleased to see him, and his attitude toward them remained paternal, as if they were indeed little children. If they appeared so, it was, of course, likely his doing.

Their relatives were less delighted. Rebecca Welch, whose mother had been operated on in 1953 for postpartum depression, claimed, "I personally think that something in Dr. Freeman wanted to be able to conquer people and take away who they were."[53] Whether or not he had these sinister intentions, this was one of the darkest chapters in American medical history. It's one that we look back on with a good deal of shame. Part of the blame lies with a midcentury zeal for conformity. People were willing to sacrifice whole personalities to make those who seemed different and unusual more like everyone else. Some who turned to lobotomies desperately yearned for a cure for their ailments; others were suffering from nothing more than human frailty. We seemed to forget that if you go around cutting up the brains of everyone who isn't "normal," by the time you are finished there will be no one left. A charismatic demagogue was elevated and trusted because he was captivating and because researching facts, as well as listening to dull doctors who have done their homework, is hard and time-consuming.

We really need to avoid behaving that way, in general.

But look, there is one thing about lobotomies—and it's the only thing, really—that makes me take heart. It's that everyone I have ever met is terrified of them. Maybe that's because of their gruesome artistic portrayals or any number of dark jokes about the procedure. Still, the fact that people now respond to the idea of being "happy but vacant" with such a primal level of horror makes me respect my fellow man.

There's a story called "Zombies" by Chuck Palahniuk. It's possibly the most Palahniuk tale ever written (readers of his work will understand). It features teenagers inflicting lobotomies on themselves. They do it so they don't have "to keep track of all three hundred Kardashian sisters and eight hundred Baldwin brothers" and can instead "be thrilled with penny candy and reruns of *Fraggle Rock*." So Chuck Palahniuk clearly has no idea in what year this story is taking place.

(The only Baldwins I can name are Ireland and Alec. That's a lie. I can name all of the Baldwins, but my head is truly a bottomless pit of useless trivia.)

No one I have ever passed this story on to has ever liked it. People have informed me that it's "scary," "horrifying," "awful, Jesus, why did you send this to me?" and, in one case, "Do you know how much DVDs of *Fraggle Rock* COST?" (A lot, apparently!) No one has ever read this story and said, "Jen, I think those teenagers had the right idea."

People don't seem to regard giving up their higher reasoning for a life of untroubled bliss as a good trade. If you want to read more into that statement, you could probably say this implies something great about humanity. Perhaps we prioritize a life of meaning over one of simple happiness. You can be happy by basically obeying all your impulses and fondling your genitals and not worrying about anything—which seems to describe the "happiness cult" that Becky and countless other less enthusiastic patients seemed to have joined. But if you want to have a meaningful life, where you take care of others, and maybe leave the world a tiny bit better than it was when you came into it, you're going to need your frontal lobes.

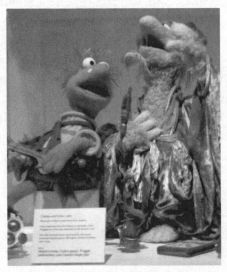

Laugh your cares away / Worries
for another day!

Polio

I don't think there is any
philosophy that suggests having
polio is a good thing.

—BILL GATES

Every so often, everyone does everything right, and humanity triumphs. The story of how we vanquished polio isn't just about Jonas Salk, although he will be remembered as a man who fought valiantly against a terrible disease. It is also an account of the greatness of people when they come together and work as a team to eradicate a true foe. In this case, we all battled polio like *soldiers*. Many people in this tale are so great and brave that you are going to want to kiss all of America-circa-1956 or give it a gruff but meaningful handshake, whichever is your preference.

The polio story is my favorite in this book.

It begins with a disease that had been terrorizing North America for fifty years. In the terrific *Polio: An American Story*, the author David M. Oshinsky explains that during the 1940s, "no disease drew as much attention, or struck the same terror, as polio. And for good reason. Polio hit without warning. There was no way of telling who would get it and who would be spared. It killed some of its victims and marked others for life, leaving behind vivid reminders for all to see: wheelchairs, crutches, leg braces, breathing devices, deformed limbs."[1] And it was common. Polio affected tens of thousands of Americans. After first appearing in the United States in the late 1890s, in 1916 there were 27,000 reported cases. The disease became an ever-present threat. In 1949 there were 40,000 cases of polio in the United States. By 1952 there were 57,879.[2] A 1952 national poll "What Americans Most Feared" listed polio as second, after the atomic bomb.[3] One reason the disease was so terrifying was that it mainly affected children under the age of five, sometimes rendering them paralyzed for life.[4]

Polio works in ways that, at first glance, seem similar to cholera. Like cholera, the virus, which is found in feces, enters through the mouth and is ingested. So, once again, it can be transmitted by unclean water. Now, you might say, "Wait. People in twentieth-century America had cesspools in their basement and were drinking unfiltered water?" Well, no. I suppose maybe some people did, but not many. The real concern was children playing in lakes, water holes, and swimming pools that at that time still used a somewhat antiquated filtration system. (Chlorine, which inactivates the polio virus, wouldn't be introduced in pools until 1946.)[5] Ingesting contaminated water from those sources *could* give you polio. Accordingly, the summer months were peak polio season; many parents were afraid to let their children go anywhere near a pool for fear they might contract the disease. Polio is one reason that the idea of someone pooping in a pool is *so* horrifying, in addition to just being very uncool. And the nitrogen in urine converts chlorine in such a way that it irritates the eyes, so stop peeing in pools, too. The latter has nothing to do with polio; just stop doing gross things in the pool because you're ruining it for everyone.

I was curious whether the reason pools were segregated at that time had to do with an insane notion that black people were more likely to carry the polio virus, but that's not the case. In fact there was a senseless stereotype at the time that black people *could not* get polio. (They can.) Pools were segregated for *different* ludicrous racist reasons that had nothing to do with disease.

In addition to swimming, someone could get polio if an infected person failed to wash their hands after going to the bathroom or changing a baby's diaper, and then prepared food. Once ingested, the virus made its way down the digestive tract and began breeding in the small intestine. From there it had the potential to attack the brain stem and central nervous system, where it could destroy nerve cells that regulate muscle control. In about one in two hundred cases, such as that of President Franklin Delano Roosevelt (FDR), paralysis resulted after the nerve cells were destroyed. The paralysis generally affected the legs. That's why we associate the disease with wheelchairs and leg braces. In some cases, with rehabilitative work, those people regained some abilities. However, in about two-thirds of cases sufferers were left with permanent muscle weakness.[6] Except for the 1994 movie hero Forrest Gump, no children in leg braces were ever magically able to run again because bullies were tormenting them or because they were in love with Robin Wright's character or because of divine intervention.

In more terrifying cases, known as bulbar polio, the brain stem is damaged, and the breathing muscles are affected. In the 1940s those sufferers would often be put in massive "iron lungs." People would be fully inserted into the tubelike contraptions, with their head left outside. These "lungs" attempted to regulate breathing by forcing air in and out of the lungs until the patients were able to breathe by themselves again. That rehabilitation could take weeks.[7] The idea of hanging out in an iron lung for even a few minutes is enough to make me feel shaky with claustrophobia, and I am certain you are not able to read in them. Oh, does that seem like a minor concern? See how it seems after being trapped in a coffinlike tube with nothing to do for weeks.

The idea of dying is also not appealing—polio was fatal in 5 to 10 percent of paralytic polio cases.

So that is the enemy people were fighting. Now let's turn to the victors.

The first hero of this story is Franklin Delano Roosevelt. The thirty-second president of the United States had been paralyzed by polio in 1921, at the age of thirty-nine, which may surprise those who think of polio as a childhood illness. While Roosevelt would dream of walking again, he was never able to do so for more than short distances, and then only with the use of braces on both his legs. Once he became president in 1933, he also became associated with the illness. In this regard, his hero-ism was kind of thrust upon him because he absolutely did *not* want to be thought of as someone who had been paralyzed. You will almost never see pictures of FDR in the wheelchair he used privately. Meanwhile, if you watch recordings of him giving speeches, you will see that he bobs his head around so much that, frankly, it seems funny by today's standards. That wasn't a tic or a weird fashion of the 1930s. It was Roosevelt's attempt to give an impression of physical vitality. His efforts are under-standable as, during his campaign, articles in magazines like *Time* claimed, "This candidate, while mentally qualified for the presidency, is utterly unfit physically."[8] As if the main duty of the U.S. president is to run a daily marathon. Still, there were many people, especially during the Depression, who believed that paralysis was a kind of moral failing and that "the world has no place for a cripple."[9]

Well, too bad, FDR, your efforts at minimizing the effects of your disease failed, and you ended up a hero to thousands of people affected by polio.

Once FDR was elected, the unfortunately widespread perception of polio victims as a drain on society began to change. Hundreds of polio survivors and parents of children with polio wrote to him. Some families told him how they had lost their life savings trying to secure appropriate medical treatment for their children. Crippled children told him how they were bullied at school because, for instance, they couldn't play baseball. He wrote back to everyone, encouraging them, telling them that they were engaged in a "brave fight," and complimenting their "fine courage and determination."[10] Some people (namely the otherwise brilliant David M. Oshinsky) say that FDR's replies were kind of glib, but you know what? He was the president of the United States, and he took time to sit down and reach out to people who were troubled. That's amazing. *The kindness of people in this troubled, sickly world is beautiful.*

One letter from a mother whose son had been paralyzed read: "Every time I hear your voice on the radio and read about your attitude toward physical handicaps—that they don't amount to a 'hill of beans'—I am strengthened and my courage is renewed. Your life is, in a way, an answer to my prayers."[11]

FDR supported a number of charities that helped polio survivors. He created the Warm Springs Foundation to benefit the Warm Springs Institute for Rehabilitation. Roosevelt had bought an estate and the surrounding twelve hundred acres in Warm Springs, Georgia, in 1926 and turned it into a veritable paradise for those suffering the aftereffects of polio. The Institute offered accessible buildings for those with disabilities and allowed them to bathe in therapeutic waters. It might seem surprising that the waters were such a huge draw, given polio's method of contagion, but for those with severely weakened muscles, swimming proved a great form of exercise. Roosevelt had stayed at Warm Springs shortly after he first contracted polio and continued to visit regularly for the rest of his life. Polio victims found it was more than simply a place to rehabilitate; it was a place where the participants could remember that they were no less human than everyone else. That was a challenge in an era when, as the disability rights activist Irving Zola noted, many felt they were "deformed, dis-eased, dis-abled, dis-ordered, ab-normal, and, most telling of all . . . in-valid."[12] Suicide was ranked the fifth-likeliest cause of death among polio victims (compared to around tenth for most Americans).[13] That's not surprising if you felt your life's prospects had been suddenly ripped away. Many adults with the disease would have to return to their childhood homes to be cared for.

Hugh Gallagher, who had contracted polio and been paralyzed during his first semester at college in 1952, was devastated by the knowledge he might never walk again. He initially had no interest in visiting Warm Springs, remarking that he did not wish "to associate with cripples."[14] He got over that, and later claimed: "Warm Springs provided an opportunity to meet people, undertake joint activities, make friends, date, fall in love. The whole range of normal social activities went on at Warm Springs, much the way it did at the rest of the world . . . Warm Springs was the best thing ever to happen to me."[15]

If Roosevelt had done nothing to help fight polio except buy and raise funds for Warm Springs, he'd have been a hero. But there's more! During his presidency, when funds for the institute seemed depleted, Roosevelt gave permission for presidential "Birthday Balls" to be held in his name on his birthday. A percentage of all ticket sales went to Warm Springs and, later, to other causes that assisted the fight against polio. The first ball was held in 1934. The publicist Carl Byoir organized the event by sending notes to newspaper editors in cities across the United States asking them to find a civic leader who would help organize a ball. Society ladies *loved* that stuff. Really, anyone would. If your town's newspaper reached out to you and said that the president hoped you would organize a party to help paralyzed children, you'd do it. You would probably head the committee.

We would order some fancy pizzas and champagne and some of those minicupcakes everybody likes. It would be great. What a good reason to have a party! Americans agreed. Six thousand Birthday Balls were held across the United States in 1934, with the slogan "We dance so that others might walk."[16] Communities attempted to outdo one another. There was a twenty-eight-foot cake and a flock of debutantes at the ball held at the Waldorf Astoria in Manhattan, but for my money the best one was hosted at Warm Springs. There the residents danced in their wheelchairs before cutting a seven-foot cake. President Roosevelt said afterward, "It was the happiest birthday I have ever known."[17]

While the balls continued until 1940, they didn't necessarily appeal to Republicans or, I suppose, people who do not like oversized cakes. "I am willing to contribute to the [polio campaign] on any day but Roosevelt's birthday"[18] became a common response from his political opponents, which would have been acceptable had they ever gotten around to donating the other 364 days of the year. So in 1938 Roosevelt established a nonpartisan group called the National Foundation for Infantile Paralysis (NFIP). Its aim was to fund promising research as well as provide the best treatment available for those afflicted by the disease. Before polio was cured, approximately two-thirds of Americans donated to the NFIP's March of Dimes fund-raiser, and 7 million volunteered on behalf of the foundation. That is a *shocking* number. That's more Americans than have volunteered for any cause that isn't related to a war.[19]

It was this foundation that helped fund Jonas Salk's research for a polio vaccine.

Jonas Salk is often remembered as the closest you can come to a secular saint in U.S. history, but he started life as a regular kid growing up in New York. Salk was born in 1914 in New York City, after his family moved to the United States from Russia to avoid persecution for their Jewish faith. That was only two years before polio epidemics would make their entrance in America;

2,343 people would die of polio in New York in 1916. Salk did not care about this problem because he was two. All you care about at age two is whether or not you can eat paste. However, Salk's mother, Dora, was very concerned about the outbreak and responded by fastidiously cleaning the apartment, making everyone remove their shoes before entering, and isolating Jonas from other children. Certainly, the fear of polio was something that influenced his upbringing, as did the threat of influenza, because the Spanish flu broke out when Jonas was four. His early life would be defined by fear of disease.

No wonder he wanted to be a doctor. Salk was something of a wunderkind and was accepted to the City College of New York at age fifteen. By age nineteen he was studying for his medical degree at the New York University (NYU) School of Medicine. He chose NYU in large part because it didn't discriminate against Jews—unlike, for instance, Yale, where the dean decreed that no more than five Jews would be accepted out of all applicants per year. (Jews had it slightly better than Irish Catholics—only two of them were allowed admittance.) Salk *loved* medical school and excelled in his studies. He recalled: "At the end of my first year of medical school, I received an opportunity to spend a year in research and teaching biochemistry. At the end of that year I was told I could, if I wished, switch and get a PhD in biochemistry but my preference was to stay with medicine. And I believe all this was linked to my original ambition, or desire, which was to be of some help to humankind."[20]

During his final year in medical school, Salk would meet his mentor, Dr. Thomas Francis, who was attempting to create a flu vaccine. Salk was exceedingly enthusiastic about this project; Dr. Francis would later note, "Dr. Salk is a member of the Jewish race but has, I believe, a very great capacity to get on with people."[21]

It may seem I am hanging a lot of Salk's story on his Jewishness, but it did have a considerable influence. By the early twentieth century society had stopped burning Jews to try to eradicate the bubonic plague, but it was still *extremely* anti-Semitic, and not just in Germany. Just as FDR's life would help alter society's perception of people with disabilities, Salk's would play a role in the United States becoming slightly more tolerant.

However, his legacy is not completely spotless. By 1942 Dr. Francis had become head of the Department of Epidemiology at the University of Michigan. He asked Salk to work in his lab because thousands of soldiers were dying of influenza and they desperately needed a vaccine. That is a noble goal. Unfortunately, it led to an extreme lapse of ethical judgment on Salk's part (which is the first thing antivaccine websites will tell you about his career). Salk participated in a study that injected institutionalized mental patients with an experimental flu vaccine without their consent. Many of them were senile and barely able to describe their symptoms. That behavior was so stupid and evil. If it makes you hate Jonas Salk, that's fine! By any modern-day ethical standard, Salk's conduct was appalling. By the standards of the *time*, it was controversial; you already know from the lobotomy chapter how badly mental patients were treated in the United States during the 1940s. Exploiting people who are already ill, and in need of help, compassion, and respect, is something that should upset people.

If you want to say you do not care for Salk and skip ahead to the other people involved in this story, that is fine. There are many! Skim right to the Eisenhower stuff! However, I am inclined to believe that the good Salk did in his life outweighs this lapse.

It is easier for me to continue liking Salk because his influenza vaccine worked. Francis and Salk developed the flu vaccine in 1938, though it's modified every year because flu strains change annually. They got lucky. If their vaccine had not worked and if the patients had died, Salk and Francis would be monsters. If it did not work and they had screamed, "It works if I say it works!" then they would be Walter Jackson Freeman II.

Feel free to start using Walter Jackson Freeman II as an insult directed toward people you hate. Almost no one will get the reference, but if I am in the room we'll high-five and it will be awesome.

Salk was celebrated for his work on the flu vaccine, and by 1947 he turned his attention to polio. The NFIP funded a lab, and Salk began researching the disease.

He began working on a killed virus vaccine. There are both live and killed virus vaccines. The purpose of all vaccines is to expose the body to a weaker version of a disease, which will cause the body to create antibodies to fight that disease. Vaccines in general act like training wheels for your immune system. Live virus vaccines expose the body to a weakened form of a virus. It's like the way people used to scratch their arms and then rub fluids or pustules from those with smallpox into the cut in order to contract a milder version of the disease, except now the process is *much* safer. In order to weaken those diseases today, we do not just crush up sick people's pustules; we generally use processes like breeding the virus in animal—generally chicken—embryos. After a virus has grown in a few embryos, it adapts to become very good at growing in chicken embryos. However, as it does so, it forgets how to grow in humans. So a human patient is injected with the chicken-embryo form of the virus. Your body sees it but kills it easily because it's a weak pathetic version of a virus that can't replicate effectively in a human. But now your immune system recognizes that virus, knows how to kill it, and can kill the full-strength virus if you're ever exposed to it again. The downside to a live virus vaccine is that in extremely rare cases, the chicken-embryo virus can mutate into a more virulent or hostile strain of the disease inside you. Mutation, it must be noted, is incredibly, statistically insignificantly unlikely, and even if it did occur, you still wouldn't become autistic or experience the other negative outcomes anti-vaccine proponents try to peddle.

Live virus vaccines are effective, but Salk wanted to develop a killed virus vaccine. A killed virus vaccine entirely inactivates a virus. Scientists can do that in a few ways, such as exposing the virus to extreme heat or formaldehyde. Therefore, some vaccines contain an extremely diluted amount of formaldehyde, which sounds scary, as formaldehyde in large doses is linked to cancer. However, formaldehyde also occurs naturally in your body and helps you metabolize food. The amount you would find in a vaccine is not even close to the amount that would be dangerous to humans. For some comparison, if this sort of thing interests you, there is a smaller trace amount of formaldehyde in a vaccine than you would find in an apple. (A vaccine contains at most 0.1 milligrams, while your average apple contains 6 milligrams.)[22]

An inactivated virus can't replicate inside you at all. And amazingly, the immune system still recognizes this inactivated virus as a danger and mounts a response against it. That's great! The downside is that the body doesn't get quite as good at fighting the virus. If you think of training your body to fight against a significantly weaker opponent with a live virus vaccine, killed virus vaccines are like training your body to fight against a dummy. Killed virus vaccines tend to provide a shorter period of immunity than live virus vaccines, which means, at least at first, that they require booster shots every few years.

In short, live virus vaccines work better on the first try, which is an advantage if you are in an area where people can't or won't come in for yearly booster shots. Killed virus vaccines are a tiny bit safer but require follow-ups.

While Salk was trying to produce a killed virus vaccine, his rival Albert Sabin, who was also funded by the NFIP to develop a polio vaccine, was trying to produce a live virus vaccine. The two would become bitter rivals, with Sabin referring to Salk as merely "a kitchen chemist."[23]

If the two were in a race, Salk won. On March 26, 1953, Salk announced on CBS radio that "it has also been shown that the amount of antibody induced by vaccination compares favorably with that which develops after natural infection." Which meant his vaccine was working.[24]

The American people heard Salk's announcement. Oh, they heard him. The *Pittsburgh Sun-Telegraph* declared: "This is not only a triumph for American medical research. It is also a triumph for every one of us who has given to the March of Dimes, which made the research possible. The dimes that we gave have produced a dividend of 1,000,000 percent or so in heart-warming experience in shared good."[25]

The only thing left to do was test the vaccine on human volunteers. In a nationwide trial of this experimental vaccine in 1954, American parents volunteered 1.8 million of their children to serve as test subjects; about 600,000 would ultimately be given either the placebo or the experimental polio vaccine. Approximately 325,000 adults—the largest group of volunteers ever assembled in the United States during peacetime—gathered to help administer the tests.[26] *Time* magazine reported: "Dr. Salk's laboratories could not produce more than a fraction of the hundreds of gallons of vaccine needed for such a massive trial. So it is being made according to his specifications on a nonprofit basis by five pharmaceutical houses—Parke, Davis & Co. in Detroit, Pitman-Moore and Eli Lilly & Co. in Indianapolis, Wyeth Inc. in Philadelphia, the Cutter Laboratories in Berkeley, Calif."[27] On *a nonprofit basis*. This is such a selfless moment in human history that it feels like one of those chapters in a science fiction series where there's a brief period of "utopia" before everyone becomes reptiles or is eaten by alien overlords.

On April 13, 1955, the *New York Times* ran a headline joyfully yelling in all caps: "SALK POLIO VACCINE PROVES SUC-

CESS; MILLIONS WILL BE IMMUNIZED SOON; CITY SCHOOLS BEGIN SHOTS APRIL 25." The article declared, "The world learned today that its hopes for finding an effective weapon against crippling polio had at last been realized."[28]

As you might expect, this was a huge deal for Salk. That same day he was asked by the CBS newsman Edward R. Murrow whether he was planning to patent the vaccine (and thereby make millions). When Murrow asked the researcher who owned the patent, Salk famously replied, "Well, the people, I would say. There is no patent. Could you patent the sun?"[29]

He gave the formula away for free.

If Salk had patented his vaccine, he would have made, depending upon how you interpret patent law, between 2.5 billion and 7 billion dollars.[30] *Can you imagine how many Wu-Tang albums he could have kept from the public with that money?* So whenever you feel cynical about whether the human race is made up of selfish jerks, remember that Jonas Salk sacrificed billions of dollars because he hoped it would prevent more children around the world from losing the ability to walk.

Full disclosure: I would have patented that vaccine and not felt guilty about it for a second. I suspect I would have used the money to do dumb stuff I thought was awesome like start an F. Scott Fitzgerald theme park. I assume everyone else would also do that. (Why doesn't a theme park devoted to books exist? It would be so much fun! Just a thought. Just what I'd do.)

Salk, however, seemed to realize that the American people, more than anyone else, were the true owners of the vaccine. After all, hadn't they danced for it, and raised money for it, and volunteered in large numbers, all to create it? Both the NFIP and the University of Pittsburgh had looked into patenting the vaccine, which Salk had no interest in doing. Now, there are many people who say that Salk couldn't have patented the vaccine even if he had wanted to because it incorporated prior medical techniques. However, the polio vaccine was viewed as such a miracle that Salk could probably have burned down the White House and everyone would have been *fine with it*. Very few Americans would have objected to him becoming a billionaire in exchange for the lives he saved. Many people were in fact outraged that Salk didn't benefit monetarily, and wrote to the president suggesting that the government give Salk "big money" and/or "lots of cash!"[31] This is one of the few times in history when people adamantly wished for someone who was not themselves to get an enormous payday. Salk did, in fact, get lots of cash. He received so many monetary gifts that an assistant at his lab said, "Paper money [went] into one bin, checks into another, and metal coins into a third."[32] He received free cars, which he donated to charities.

He also earned acclaim that no money could buy. Publications across the country celebrated him, with articles like the one in *Newsweek* declaring the polio vaccine "A Quiet Young Man's Magnificent Victory." Movie studios wanted to share his life story; Salk suggested that it would be better for them to wait until he was dead.

President Dwight D. Eisenhower met with Salk in the White House Rose Garden on April 22, 1955. There Eisenhower promised to give Salk's vaccine to "every country that welcomed the knowledge, including the Soviet Union." (The Soviet Union! During the Cold War!) He declared Salk a "benefactor to mankind."[33] Before handing Salk a special citation, honoring his achievement, Eisenhower said:

> When I think of the countless thousands of American parents and grandparents who are hereafter to be spared the agonizing fears of the annual epidemic of poliomyelitis, when I think of all the agony that these people will be spared seeing their loved ones suffering in bed, I must say to you I have no words in which adequately to express the thanks of myself and all the people I know—all 164 million Americans, to say

nothing of all the people in the world that will profit from your discovery. I am very, very happy to hand this to you.[34]

Salk gave a self-deprecating response claiming that it had really been a group effort.

Now that the vaccine existed, the next challenge was how to distribute it to everyone.

On May 21, 1955, President Eisenhower declared that the polio vaccine was currently being screened and would be released within a few days. He explained the vaccination programs that would be in place for children:

> Since April 12 the National Foundation for Infantile Paralysis has been furnishing free vaccine for children in the first and second grades, and for children in the third grade who participated in the field tests of vaccine last year. [Millions of] children have been vaccinated—including one of my grandchildren, a first grader. This free vaccination program is the initial method for getting the vaccine to our children. No vaccine is now being distributed in any other way . . .
>
> To assure that no child is denied vaccination by reason of its cost, some states and localities may operate mass free public vaccination programs for all children. Other States may provide free vaccination only for children whose parents are unable to pay, through clinics, schools and preschool programs, or by furnishing free vaccine to private physicians. In those States, a portion of the State allocation of vaccine will flow into normal drug distribution channels for the exclusive use of children in the priority age brackets— to be administered by family doctors.
>
> To assist the States in providing free vaccinations, I have recommended that the Congress enact legislation making $28 million available to the States for the purchase of vaccine. This legislation is now being considered by the appropriate

Committees of the Congress and I urge its immediate adoption.[35]

It is notable that a famous Republican war hero president was desperately urging the American people to make free medical treatment available to its citizens. Do you like to discuss politics? If so, this fact may be useful to you someday.

By encouraging the community to be vaccinated—and trying to limit the expense of doing so—Eisenhower wasn't just providing peace of mind to millions of families. He was also increasing herd immunity among the population. The herd immunity theory, which shows up as early as 1900 in the *Lancet*, is the premise that outbreaks of diseases like polio "arose because of the accrual of a critical number of susceptible individuals in populations and that epidemics could be delayed or averted by maintaining numbers of susceptible individuals below this critical density (i.e, by maintaining the proportion of immune above some threshold)."[36] Basically, if a large majority of the population is immunized, even if you are a fool who refuses to vaccinate your children, it is still unlikely they will contract measles or mumps or polio because most of the rest of society is vaccinated. To which you might say, "Jennifer, I love being a murderous idiot. Why should I vaccinate my children if they probably won't get a disease anyway, because everyone else cares about their children's health and vaccinated them accordingly?" Well, herd immunity works for most diseases only if about 80 to 90 percent of the population is vaccinated. With some diseases, like measles, a 95 percent vaccination rate is necessary. So if enough people decide that their yoga teacher is really onto something and they are not going to immunize their kids, because they are going to feed them a whole bunch of grapes instead, then the number of immunized people drops beneath the percentage necessary for herd immunity to be effective. That sounds ridiculous because clearly most people vaccinate their kids, right?

Well, Zimbabwe now has a higher immunization rate for one-year-olds against measles (around 95 percent) than the United States does. So do 112 other countries, according to the World Health Organization (WHO).[37] We are down to a 91 percent vaccination rate for measles, which, according to the WHO, makes us much more vulnerable to outbreaks. That is why, for instance, there was an outbreak at Disneyland in 2014. This is very bad news for people in the United States who are especially vulnerable to diseases, including those with compromised immune systems or babies who are too young to be vaccinated.

Refusing to vaccinate puts at risk not just your children but the people in our communities who most require our protection. This is a substantial downside for people deciding to protect their kids via star signs and "good vibes" instead of medicine. (Horoscopes are, to be fair, a lot of fun.)

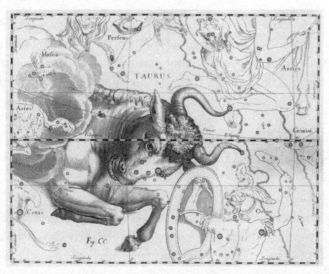

I'm a Taurus! One of our personality traits is not believing horoscopes are real!

Nobody wanted people to be at risk for polio. Not Eisenhower, not Salk, not the people who had lived so long in fear of the disease. Most people were vaccinated immediately. Unfortunately, there were some mishaps. Two batches of vaccine produced at the Cutter laboratories in California did not sufficiently kill the virus, which resulted in the deaths of ten children. This wasn't Salk's fault. His vaccine worked. It was the fault of the laboratory. (It used a glass filter rather than an asbestos one when trying to kill the virus, which allowed some of the live virus to seep through.) This incident led to increased federal regulations of vaccines and "better procedures for filtration, storage, and safety testing were developed."[38] In 1955 there were 10 regulators overseeing vaccines employed by the National Institutes of Health. By 1956 there were 150. Today the Food and Drug Administration (FDA) employs 250 people to monitor the production of every vaccine to ensure that there is never a repeat of the Cutter incident. Vaccines are tested tens of thousands of times to ensure they contain exactly what is represented.[39]

Whew. Good.

Polio was effectively eliminated throughout the world. And then people just . . . kind of forgot all about polio. This seems to be the human response to any disease. People forget diseases ever existed the *minute* they are no longer being affected by them. Maybe that's understandable. Maybe if we all thought about all the potential diseases the world is teeming with, and the extent to which we are, every day, dancing on the edge of a volcano, the world would seem too terrifying to walk around in at all.

Or we'd just vaccinate our kids.

"Our main problem now," said Thomas Rivers, a leader in viral research who oversaw the clinical trials of Salk's vaccine in 1956, "is not that anything is wrong with the Salk vaccine, but that something is wrong with the people who won't take it."[40] People were not necessarily apathetic or foolish. Some of their difficulties stemmed from the fact that three shots a year were required and one booster shot annually for years following. Although efforts had been made to keep the polio vaccine extremely affordable, visiting doctors still costs money. And people living in rural areas far away from a local doctor sometimes couldn't afford the time to make that many trips, especially since the situation no longer seemed dire.

In 1961 Albert Sabin's vaccine became available. The American Medical Association recommended that Sabin's live virus vaccine replace Salk's killed virus vaccine. Sabin's vaccine could be taken orally—sometimes hidden in a sugar cube—and once taken, it provided lasting immunity. It does cause polio in very rare cases (one in 2.7 million).[41] That said, it's cheaper to manufacture, which is an advantage. By 1963 it was the vaccine of choice, and Sabin became the new face of the polio fight, although he was never as beloved as Salk.

For some time afterward Salk's vaccine was forgotten. This haunted Salk for the rest of his life. He *hated* Sabin's vaccine. The rivalry and enduring dislike between the two scientists is well documented and would make for a really great movie if anyone wants to produce it.

Today, Salk's vaccine is used primarily in the United States and Europe, while Sabin's is more popular in periphery countries. I'd like to say that today Salk and Sabin could take pride in knowing that both vaccines are used, though they really hated each other, so that might be a bit optimistic.

Salk never stopped trying to be of "some help to humankind." In 1962 he founded the Salk Institute for Biological Studies in La Jolla, California, which he hoped would serve as "a cathedral to science." The competition to work there was so steep that Salk joked, "I couldn't possibly have become a member of this institute if I hadn't founded it myself."[42] Salk continued to work until he died of heart failure in 1993. During the last years of his life he devoted his attention to finding a vaccine for AIDS.

He said he knew that many people expected him to fail in his attempts, but he maintained, "There is no such thing as failure. You can only fail if you stop too soon."[43] He never did develop that vaccine, maybe simply because death stopped him. But he never gave up. And he never stopped believing in the fundamental capacity for goodness in people. "What is important is that we, Number one: Learn to live with each other," he said in 1985. "Number two: Try to bring out the best in each other. The best from the best, and the best from those who, perhaps, might not have the same endowment . . . the object is not to put down the other, but to raise up the other."[44]

Sometimes, as we go about our lives, we're angry, or other people are angry. We're idiots, or they are. Maybe it seems a lot to expect that we can lift up our fellow man and bring out the best in everyone. But we've done it before. We can work miracles when we come together to help one another. Just look at how we all cured polio.

Epilogue

Sometimes people ask me when I believe America is due for another plague. I invariably reply, "Well, we literally just had one." People who talk about the possibility of a pandemic that kills millions as though it is somehow unlikely seem to forget that. Perhaps that's because it just didn't look like what television shows about plagues depict. There were no government officials in hazmat suits sweeping into neighborhoods to quarantine people during our last plague. But then, as we've seen, the response to plagues rarely looks like that. People, more than anything, want to go about life as normal, even during a plague.

But AIDs is not less horrific for that.

Indeed, the shadow of the mishandling of the AIDS crisis hangs over this entire book.

I did not want to write a chapter on AIDS. That is because I think it is my role to tell the stories of people who are already

260 🐿 **Get Well Soon**

dead and cannot speak for themselves. You may have lived through the AIDS epidemic of the 1980s yourself. If not, you know someone who did. I am certain that individuals can tell the story of those terrible times much better than I.

That said, I must conclude this book by writing at least a little about the extent to which AIDS was mishandled, because this plague seems a perfect case in point of what happens if you ignore every single one of history's lessons regarding disease.

Let's look at some of those lessons.

One of the interesting takeaways from both the Antonine plague and polio is what a difference a strong leader can make during an epidemic. Marcus Aurelius's swift response to the Antonine plague—and his attempt to help cover expenses for the general populace and rebuild the parts of the army decimated by the disease—staved off the fall of the Roman Empire, at least temporarily. When FDR took up polio as a cause, America followed his lead and went to work eradicating it. Although his role may not have been as significant, Eisenhower is also to be commended for trying to ensure that cost did not prohibit any child from receiving the polio vaccine, and that the vaccine was shared with the world. Those men each acknowledged the seriousness of their crises and went about bravely confronting the disease in their midst head-on. They did not ignore it or glamorize it or shame people for having it, because *that never works*. That strategy just gives diseases more time to multiply and kill people. Diseases are *delighted* when you refuse to take them seriously.

When members of the Ronald Reagan administration first heard about AIDS, they laughed about the blossoming epidemic. Mark Joseph Stern described the infamous episode in this *Slate* account:

On October 15, 1982, at a White House press briefing, reporter Lester Kinsolving asked press secretary Larry Speakes about

a horrifying new disease called AIDS that was ravaging the
gay community.

"What's AIDS?" Speakes asked.

"It's known as the 'gay plague,'" Kinsolving replied.

Everyone laughed.

"I don't have it," Speakes replied. "Do you?"

The room erupted in laughter again. Speakes continued
to parry Kinsolving's questions with quips, joking that Kinsolving himself might be gay simply because he knew about
the disease. The press secretary eventually acknowledged
that nobody in the White House, including Reagan, knew
anything about the epidemic.

"There has been no personal experience here," Speakes
cracked. The room was in stitches.[1]

After those in the administration had a good laugh, they
proceeded to, at least publicly, ignore AIDS. President Reagan
didn't address the disease in any capacity until September 17,
1985. When a reporter asked him about the terrifying spread of
the disease, Reagan replied:

We have $100 million in the budget this year; it'll be
$126 million next year. So, this is a top priority with us. Yes,
there's no question about the seriousness of this and the need
to find an answer.

Q: If I could follow up, sir. The scientist who talked
about this, who does work for the Government, is in the
National Cancer Institute. He was referring to your program
and the increase that you proposed as being not nearly enough
at this stage to go forward and really attack the problem.

The President: I think with our budgetary constraints and all,
it seems to me that $126 million in a single year for research
has got to be something of a vital contribution.[2]

In reality, Reagan slashed the AIDS budget by 11 percent in 1986. It went from $95 to $85.5 million.[3]

The president did not hold a major public address to discuss the disease until 1987, after 20,849 Americans had already died of it. The Gay Men's Health Crisis was founded in 1981. *An Early Frost* appeared on television in 1985. *The Normal Heart* was staged at the Public Theater in New York by 1985. The actor Rock Hudson would die that same year. The surgeon general was sending reports endorsing condom usage in 1986. *What was Reagan waiting for?*

I do not know if medical progress on the disease could have been accelerated. But I certainly know that a leader can change the way the public *responds* to an outbreak of disease. Reagan was called "the great communicator." He was, perhaps, one of our most charismatic presidents. He was *beloved*, and he was personally friendly with gay people. Imagine what it would have meant, right from the beginning, to have had a leader who said, "Americans do not let other Americans be struck down in the prime of their lives by a plague. It doesn't matter who they are or how they live their lives. We are a courageous people, and we are going to come together to fight this dreadful disease."

I am always trying to rewrite the scripts for history, the way some people must mentally rewrite the scripts for disappointing episodes of their favorite television shows. I admit I have not succeeded in changing anything, yet.

A more compassionate, humane response might not have halted the spread of the AIDS epidemic, but it surely would have been better than laughing at it.

By 1987 the prominent conservative William F. Buckley Jr. suggested that everyone with AIDS should be "tattooed in the upper forearm, to protect common-needle users, and on the buttocks, to prevent the victimization of other homosexuals."[4]

This stance had nothing on California congressman William

Dannemeyer's statement that if he could identify everyone with AIDS, he would respond by "wip[ing] them off the face of the earth."[5] The Arkansas senator and later governor Mike Huckabee took an infinitesimally more moderate view in 1992: "It is the first time in the history of civilization in which carriers of a genuine plague have not been isolated from the general population . . . we need to take steps that would isolate the carriers of the plague."[6] We keep considering this man as a presidential candidate, and he basically said that everyone with AIDS should be rounded up and shipped off to an island.

Whenever someone casually refers to "the history of civilization" in a way that does not jibe with the history of civilization as I extensively, constantly, read about it, I like to research their favorite books to see where they are getting their information. In most of these cases all their favorite books have titles like *Christmas, Guns, and Integrity.*

Huckabee's statement was ill informed. As you know from reading this book, it is not the first time in civilization that carriers of a plague were not forced into isolation. It seems most likely he was thinking of lepers, and in that case *quarantine wasn't a good thing.* It was a disaster. The nightmarish conditions on the island of Molokai required a man of Father Damien's rare compassion and courage to bring order and welfare. And that disease wasn't even especially contagious.

Meanwhile, carriers of the highly contagious tuberculosis were off at the opera and hunting alligators for fun and profit. It is telling that, historically, quarantines extended primarily to those who had less wealth, power, and social clout.

In instances during the AIDS epidemic when nonsufferers—modern-day Father Damiens—came together to rally for more federal funding for AIDS, Huckabee complained: "An alternative would be to request that multimillionaire celebrities, such as Elizabeth Taylor . . . Madonna and others who are pushing for more AIDS funding be encouraged to give out of their own personal treasuries increased amounts for AIDS research."[7] It is worth noting that the bulk of proceeds from the auction of Taylor's $150 million jewelry collection did indeed go to AIDS research.[8] So in the end she gave about as much as the government did in 1986. That said, relying on a single woman, even one as generous and generally magnificent as Elizabeth Taylor, to take care of a national health crisis is not realistic.

Of course, government representatives and wealthy celebrities aren't the only ones who can make a difference when it comes to the fight against disease. By looking to Father Damien's treatment of the lepers, or Reverend Henry Whitehead's support of John Snow's cholera research, we can see the difference religious figures can make. Perhaps it seems only natural that they, more than anyone else, would devote themselves to relieving the pain of those suffering. But during the AIDS crisis the religious right claimed that homosexuals should burn in hell and that the disease was God's punishment. The popular pastor Billy Graham pondered before an audience, "Is AIDS a judgment of God? I could not say for sure, but I think so."[9]

Graham, I am pleased to say, at least eventually apologized for this statement. The Reverend Walter Alexander, of Reno's First Baptist Church, who stated that, to combat the epidemic, "we should do what the Bible says and cut their throats,"[10] did not. In 1989 Catholic bishops *strongly* objected to the use of condoms specifically to stop the spread of AIDS.[11] This stance was, obviously, both dumb and deadly.

I am sure there were religious groups that were kind and compassionate and behaved in a Christian fashion. I would love to hear stories about the pastors and priests and others drawn to religion because they wished to help their fellow men. I know there must have been many who helped fight this scourge. I am certain they exist. But they do get overshadowed by the "Burn in hell, fags" signs from this period. I suppose God could be an intolerant God. I have never met God. But if he is as cruel as these people made him out to be, then, like that sixteenth-century Cuban, I'd rather take my chances in hell with the devil.

The stigma around AIDS rivaled that around syphilis. Remember that character who said that you wouldn't even want to share a room with someone with syphilis, let alone shake hands with him? People were equally afraid to touch people with AIDS, likely because it took a monstrously long time to get information on how the disease actually spread. As late as 1985, Reagan wasn't exactly sure whether children with AIDS should be in schools.

In some cases, even the families of those with AIDS forsook them. Ruth Coker Burks, who cared for thousands of people dying of AIDS, recalled in *The Arkansas Times* the number of families who abandoned their children in the early days of the epidemic. She recalled her first experience calling a mother who hung up on her:

> "I called her back," Burks said. "I said, 'If you hang up on me again, I will put your son's obituary in your hometown newspaper and I will list his cause of death.' Then I had her attention."
>
> Her son was a sinner, the woman told Burks. She didn't know what was wrong with him and didn't care. She wouldn't come [to see him], as he was already dead to her as far as she was concerned. She said she wouldn't even claim his body when he died. It was a curse Burks would hear again and again over the next decade: sure judgment and yawning hell-fire, abandonment on a platter of scripture. Burks estimates she worked with more than 1,000 people dying of AIDS over the years. Of those, she said, only a handful of families didn't turn their backs on their loved ones.

Burks hung up the phone, trying to decide what she should tell the dying man. "I went back in his room," she said, "and when I walked in, he said, 'Oh, momma. I knew you'd come,' and then he lifted his hand. And what was I going to do? So I took his hand. I said, 'I'm here, honey. I'm here.'"[12]

This parental rejection reminds me of the children dying of bubonic plague who cried: "Father, why have you abandoned me? Do you forget I am your child? O, Mother, where have you gone? Why are you now so cruel to me when yesterday you were so kind? You fed me at your breast and carried me within your womb for nine months." But at least parents during that earlier plague did not feel righteous about abandoning their children.

Those who had AIDS survived because they, like Mr. Crumpton's No Nose'd Club for syphilitics, founded groups like the Gay Men's Health Crisis and ACT UP to fight for their right to live. They supported one another. They protested. They yelled. They made people extremely uncomfortable.

Good for them.

There should be a statue to the leaders of those groups who fought to exist in a time of almost unrivaled hatred and foolishness in the United States.

The horrible mismanagement of the AIDS crisis makes me want to grab those people by the shoulders and shake them and say, "Why haven't you read about what worked or did not work every time a plague cropped up before this one? Why aren't you paying attention? Do not do the same stupid stuff people did before! We know what works and what doesn't! Be smarter, please, please, be smarter, be kinder, be kinder and smarter, I am begging you."

I find the forgetfulness of people, especially in true matters of life and death, so frustrating. Sometimes I look at these histories and think, *People are just going to keep making the same dumb mistakes every single time. And one day those mistakes will doom us all.*

And I feel sad and furious and frightened for what will happen next.

But then I think about how polio is almost eradicated. Or that penicillin exists. And I remember that we are progressing, always, even if that progress is sometimes slower and more uneven than we might wish. I remind myself, too, of all the ways people have persevered and survived in conditions that are surely as bad as anything that is to come.

Whenever I am most disillusioned, I look to one of my favorite quotes from *The World of Yesterday* (1942) by Stefan Zweig. When Zweig was fleeing from the Nazis and living in exile he wrote: "Even from the abyss of horror in which we try to find our way today, half-blind, our hearts distraught and shattered, I look up again to the ancient constellations of my childhood, comforting myself that, some day, this relapse will appear only an interval in the eternal rhythm of progress onward and upward."[13] I have to believe that the missteps are only intermittent relapses as we grow stronger and smarter and better. We do get better. At everything. Combatting diseases fits somewhere among "everything."

I believe there will be a day when we will see diseases as what they are—an enemy of all of humanity. Not of perceived sinners, not of people who are poor or have a different sexual orientation, not of those who we somehow decided "have it coming" because they're "not like us." Diseases are at war with all of us. Diseases don't care about any of the labels, so it makes no sense for us to.

I believe we will become more compassionate. I believe we will fight smarter. I believe that in the deepest place of our souls, we are not cowardly or hateful or cruel to our neighbors. I believe we are kind and smart and brave. I believe that as long as we follow those instincts and do not give in to terror and blame, we can triumph over diseases and the stigmas attached to them. When we fight plagues, not each other, we will not only defeat diseases but preserve our humanity in the process.

Onward and upward.

Absolutely Horrific Pictures (for Those Who Want Them) of the Effects of the Diseases

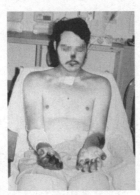

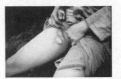

A bubo from bubonic
plague

A man suffering from
bubonic plague

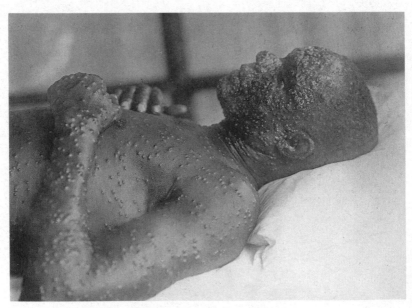

A man with smallpox

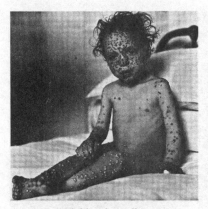

A child with smallpox

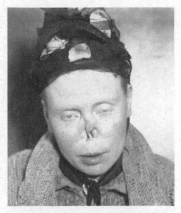

A woman with syphilis

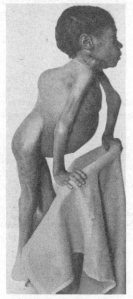

A child with tuberculosis

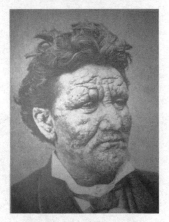

A man with leprosy

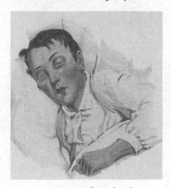

A man with typhoid

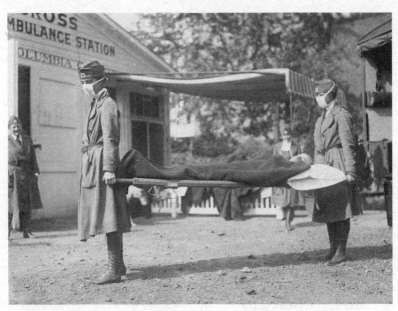

Nurses at work during the Spanish Flu

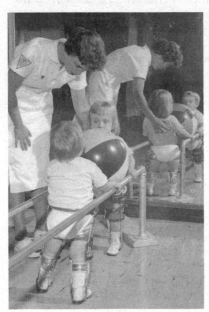

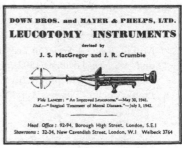

DOWN BROS. and MAYER & PHELPS, LTD.
LEUCOTOMY INSTRUMENTS
devised by

J. S. MacGregor and J. R. Crumbie

Vide LANCET: "An Improved Leucotome."—May 30, 1941.
Ibid.—"Surgical Treatment of Mental Diseases."—July 5, 1942.

Head Office : 92-94, Borough High Street, London, S.E.1
Showrooms : 32-34, New Cavendish Street, London, W.1   Welbeck 3764

The tool inserted into patients'
skulls during a lobotomy

Children exercising their limbs after polio

Notes

Antonine Plague

1. Walter Scheidel, "Marriage, Families, and Survival in the Roman Imperial Army: Demographic Aspects," Princeton/Stanford Working Papers in Classics, Stanford University, 2005, https://www.princeton.edu/~pswpc/pdfs/scheidel/110509.pdf.
2. Kathryn Hinds, *Everyday Life in the Roman Empire* (New York: Cavendish Square, 2009), p. 114.
3. Oliver J. Thatcher, *The Library of Original Sources*, vol. 4, *Early Mediaeval Age* (1901); reprint, Honolulu: University Press of the Pacific, 2004), p. 168.
4. "Germanic Peoples," *Encyclopedia Britannica*, http://www.britannica.com/topic/Germanic-peoples.
5. John George Sheppard, *The Fall of Rome and the Rise of the New Nationalities: A Series of Lectures on the Connections Between Ancient and Modern History* (1892), University of Toronto, Robarts Library archives, p. 173, https://archive.org/details/fallofromeriseof00shepuoft.
6. Frank McLynn, *Marcus Aurelius: A Life* (Cambridge, MA: Da Capo Press, 2009), p. 459.
7. Dideri Raoult and Michael Drancourt, eds., *Paleomicrobiology: Past Human Infections* (Berlin: Springer Verlag, 2008), p. 11.
8. Thucydides, *History of the Peloponnesian War*, translated by Richard Crawley (New York: Dutton, 1910), p. 132.
9. Raoult, *Paleomicrobiology*, p. 11.
10. Ibid., p. 10.
11. McLynn, *Marcus Aurelius*, p. 467.
12. Marcus Aurelius, *The Meditations of Marcus Aurelius Antoninus*, edited by A. S. L. Farquharson (Oxford: Oxford University Press [Oxford World's Classics], 2008), p. 10.
13. Brigitte Maire, ed., *"Greek" and "Roman" in Latin Medical Texts: Studies in Cultural Change and Exchange in Ancient Medicine* (Leiden: Brill, 2014), p. 235.

14. William Byron Forbush, ed., *Foxe's Book of Martyrs: A History of the Lives, Sufferings and Triumphant Deaths of the Early Christian and Protestant Martyrs* (Philadelphia: John C. Winston, 1926), "The Fourth Persecution."
15. Anthony R. Birley, *Marcus Aurelius: A Biography* (New York: Routledge, 2000), p. 159.
16. Arthur Edward Romilly Boak, *A History of Rome to 565 AD* (New York: Macmillan, 1921), Kindle edition, p. 299.
17. Marcus Tullius Cicero, *The Orations of Marcus Tullius Cicero*, translated by C. D. Young (1851), University of Toronto, Robarts Library archives, p. 162.
18. McLynn, *Marcus Aurelius*, p. 349.
19. Barthold Georg Niebuhr, *Lectures on the History of Rome: From the First Punic War to the Death of Constantine* (1844), e-source courtesy of Getty Research Institute, p. 253, https://archive.org/details/history ofrome01nieb.
20. George Childs Kohn, ed., *Encyclopedia of Plague and Pestilence: From Ancient Times to the Present*, 3rd ed. (New York: Facts on File, 2008), p. 10.
21. Edward Gibbon, *The History of the Decline and Fall of the Roman Empire* (New York: Dutton, 1910), p. 134.
22. Cassius Dio, *Roman History*, Loeb Classical Library (Cambridge, MA: Harvard University Press, 1911), p. 73.
23. Ibid.

Bubonic Plague

1. John Aberth, *From the Brink of the Apocalypse: Confronting Famine, War, Plague and Death in the Later Middle Ages* (London: Routledge, 2001), p. 112.
   Robert S. Gottfried, *The Black Death: Natural and Human Disaster in Medieval Europe* (New York: Free Press, 1983), p. 115.
2. Terry Deary, *Horrible History: The Measly Middle Ages* (New York: Scholastic, 2015), p. 36.
3. "Newcomers Facts," National Geographic Channel, October 25, 2013, http://channel.nationalgeographic.com/meltdown/articles/newcomers -facts/.
4. Gottfried, *The Black Death*, p. 135.
5. Aberth, *From the Brink of the Apocalypse*, p. 121.
6. "Myths About Onion," National Onion Association website, http://www .onions-usa.org/faqs/onion-flu-cut-myths.
7. Aberth, *From the Brink of the Apocalypse*, p. 116; Stuart A. Kallen, *Prophecies and Soothsayers (The Mysterious & Unknown)* (San Diego: Reference Point Press, 2011), p. 40.
8. John Kelly, *The Great Mortality* (New York: Harper Collins, 2005), Kindle edition, Kindle location 3791.

9. Giovanni Boccaccio, *The Decameron*, translated by John Payne (New York: Walter J. Black, 2007), Project Gutenberg e-book, https://www.gutenberg.org/files/23700/23700-h/23700-h.htm, p. 2.
10. Ibid.
11. Louise Chipley Slavicek, *Great Historic Disasters: The Black Death* (New York: Chelsea House, 2008), p. 62.
12. Kelly, *The Great Mortality*, Kindle location 2975.
13. Ibid., Kindle location 1832.
14. Ibid., Kindle location 1835.
15. Ibid., Kindle location 1826.
16. Slavicek, *Great Historic Disasters*, p. 51.
17. Boccaccio, *The Decameron*, p. 17.
18. "Medieval British History in Honor of Barbara Hannawalt," *History: The Journal of the Historical Association*, 96, no. 324 (September 9, 2011): 281, http://onlinelibrary.wiley.com/doi/10.1111/j.1468-229X.2011.00531_2.x/abstract.
19. Ibid.
20. Kelly, *The Great Mortality*, Kindle location 2981–83.
21. Slavicek, *Great Historic Disasters*, p. 51.
22. Francis Gasquet, *The Black Death of 1348 and 1349* (London: George Bell and Sons, 1908), p. 33.
23. Terry Haydn and Christine Counsell, eds., *History, ICT and Learning in the Secondary School* (London: Routledge, 2003), p. 247.
24. James Leasor, *The Plague and the Fire* (Thirsk: House of Stratus, 2001), p. 112.
25. Ibid.
26. Ronald Hans Pahl, *Creative Ways to Teach the Mysteries of History*, vol. 1 (Lanham, MD: Rowman and Littlefield Education, 2005), p. 40.
27. Ian Wilson, *Nostradamus: The Man Behind the Prophecies* (New York: St. Martin's Press, 2002), p. 45.
28. "Nostradamus Biography," the Biography.com website, http://www.biography.com/people/nostradamus-9425407#studies.
29. Boccaccio, "Day: The First," paragraph 3.
30. "Nostradamus," *Encyclopedia of World Biography*, http://www.notablebiographies.com/Ni-Pe/Nostradamus.html.
31. Diane Bailey, *The Plague (Epidemics and Society)* (New York: Rosen, 2010), p. 6; Kallen, *Prophecies and Soothsayers*, p. 45; Scarlett Ross, *Nostradamus for Dummies* (Hoboken, NJ: Wiley, 2005), p. 47.
32. Kallen, *Prophecies and Soothsayers*, p. 40; Russell Roberts, *The Life and Times of Nostradamus* (Hockessin, IN: Mitchell Lane, 2008), p. 22.
33. Kallen, *Prophecies and Soothsayers*, p. 40; Ross, *Nostradamus for Dummies*, p. 47.
34. Wilson, *Nostradamus*, p. 80.

35. "Plague—Fact Sheet No. 267," World Health Organization media website, November 2014, http://www.who.int/mediacentre/factsheets/fs267/en/.
36. "Rat-Shit-Covered Physicians Baffled by Spread of Black Plague," *Onion*, December 15, 2009, http://www.theonion.com/article/rat-shit-covered-physicians-baffled-by-spread-of-b-2876.
37. Kelly, *The Great Mortality*, Kindle location 1775.

Dancing Plague

1. John Waller, *The Dancing Plague: The Strange, True Story of an Extraordinary Illness* (Naperville, IL: Sourcebooks, 2009), p. 25.
2. Ibid.
3. E. Louis Backman, *Religious Dances*, translated by E. Classen (Alton, UK: Dance Books, 2009), p. 25.
4. Paracelsus, *Essential Theoretical Writings*, edited by Wouter J. Hanegraaff, translated by Andrew Weeks (Leiden: Brill, 2008), p. 779, http://selfdefinition.org/magic/Paracelsus-Essential-Theoretical-Writings.pdf.
5. Ibid.
6. Waller, *The Dancing Plague*, p. 17.
7. Scott Mendelson, "Conversion Disorder and Mass Hysteria," *Huffpost Healthy Living*, February 2, 2012, http://www.huffingtonpost.com/scott-mendelson-md/mass-hysteria_b_1239012.html.
8. Fred K. Berger, "Conversion Disorder," Medline Plus, October 31, 2014, https://www.nlm.nih.gov/medlineplus/ency/article/000954.htm.
9. Heinrich Kramer and James (Jacob) Sprenger, *Malleus Maleficarum* (1486), translated by Montague Summers (1928; Digireads.com, 2009), pp. 36 and 54.
10. Ibid., p. 36.
11. Waller, *The Dancing Plague*, p. 107.
12. Ibid.
13. John C. Waller, "In a Spin: The Mysterious Dancing Epidemic of 1518," *Science Direct*, September 2008, http://www.sciencedirect.com/science/article/pii/S0160932708000379.
14. John Waller, "In a Spin, the Mysterious Dancing Epidemic of 1518," Department of History, Michigan State University, East Grand River, East Lansing, MI, July 7, 2008.
15. Waller, *The Dancing Plague*, p. 21.
16. Waller, "In a Spin," http://www.sciencedirect.com/science/article/pii/S0160932708000379.
17. Waller, *The Dancing Plague*, p. 133.
18. Ibid.
19. "St. Vitus Dance," BBC Radio 3, September 7, 2012, http://www.bbc.co.uk/programmes/b018h8kv.
20. Waller, *The Dancing Plague*, p. 146.

21. H. C. Erik Midelfort, *A History of Madness in Sixteenth-Century Germany* (Stanford: Stanford University Press, 1999), p. 35.
22. Ibid.
23. Ibid., p. 36.
24. Waller, *The Dancing Plague*, p. 176.
25. Ibid., p. 180.
26. Lee Siegel, "Cambodians' Vision Loss Linked to War Trauma," *Los Angeles Times*, October 15, 1989, http://articles.latimes.com/1989-10-15/news/mn-232_1_vision-loss.
27. Simone Sebastian, "Examining 1962's 'Laughter Epidemic,'" *Chicago Tribune*, July 29, 2003, http://articles.chicagotribune.com/2003-07-29/features/0307290281_1_laughing-40th-anniversary-village.
28. "Contagious Laughter," WYNC RadioLab, Season 4, Episode 1, http://www.radiolab.org/story/91595-contagious-laughter/.
29. Waller, *The Dancing Plague*, p. 227.
30. Susan Dominus, "What Happened to the Girls in Le Roy," *New York Times Magazine*, March 7, 2012, http://www.nytimes.com/2012/03/11/magazine/teenage-girls-twitching-le-roy.html.
31. Ibid.
32. Ibid.

Smallpox

1. Jared M. Diamond, *Guns, Germs and Steel: The Fates of Human Societies* (New York: Norton, 1997), p. 70.
2. Kim MacQuarrie, *The Last Days of the Incas* (New York: Simon and Schuster, 2007), p. 111.
3. Michael Wood, *Conquistadors*, BBC Digital, 2015, https://books.google.com/books?id=xKqFCAAAQBAJ&pg=PA90&lpg=PA90&dq=%22Cort%C3%A9s+stared+at+him+for+a+moment+and+then+patted+him+on+the+head.%22&source=bl&ots=eTKqshNJKf&sig=gtnbajA3wRSChgmOFWsJgRTdGPc&hl=en&sa=X&ved=0CCYQ6AEwAWoVChMIivn7vODlxgIV1FmICh3E5QPM#v=onepage&q=smallpox&f=false, p. 122.
4. Christopher Buckley, *But Enough About You* (New York: Simon and Schuster, 2014), p. 101.
5. John Campbell, *An Account of the Spanish Settlements in America* (1762), Hathi Trust Digital Library, http://catalog.hathitrust.org/Record/008394522, p. 30.
6. Diamond, *Guns, Germs and Steel*, p. 75.
7. Ibid., p. 71.
8. Charles C. Mann, "1491," *Atlantic*, March 2002, http://www.theatlantic.com/magazine/archive/2002/03/1491/302445/.
9. Heather Pringle, "Lofty Ambitions of the Inca," *National Geographic*, April 2011, http://ngm.nationalgeographic.com/2011/04/inca-empire/pringle-text/1.

10. Wood, *Conquistadors*, p. 144.
11. Liesl Clark, "The Sacrificial Ceremony," NOVA, November 24, 1998, http://www.pbs.org/wgbh/nova/ancient/sacrificial-ceremony.html.
12. Paul Jongko, "10 Ancient Cultures That Practiced Ritual Human Sacrifice," TopTenz website, July 29, 2014, http://www.toptenz.net/10-ancient-cultures-practiced-ritual-human-sacrifice.php.
13. Wood, *Conquistadors*, p. 80.
14. Ibid., p. 82.
15. Robert I. Rotberg, ed., *Health and Disease in Human History, A Journal of Interdisciplinary History Reader* (Cambridge, MA: MIT Press, 1953), p. 198.
16. "The Story of . . . Smallpox—and Other Deadly Eurasian Germs," from *Guns, Germs and Steel*, PBS.org, http://www.pbs.org/gunsgermssteel/variables/smallpox.html.
17. Hanne Jakobsen, "The Epidemic That Was Wiped Out," *ScienceNordic*, April 14, 2012, http://sciencenordic.com/epidemic-was-wiped-out.
18. Gerald N. Grob, *The Deadly Truth: A History of Disease in America* (Cambridge, MA: Harvard University Press, 2005), p. 31.
19. Noble David Cook, *Born to Die: Disease and New World Conquest, 1492–1650* (Cambridge: Cambridge University Press, 1998), p. 66.
20. Rotberg, *Health and Diseases*, p. 198.
21. Wood, *Conquistadors*, p. 127.
22. "The Conquest of the Incas—Francisco Pizarro," PBS.org, http://www.pbs.org/conquistadors/pizarro/pizarro_flat.html.
23. MacQuarrie, *The Last Days of the Incas*, p. 69.
24. Heather Whipps, "How Smallpox Changed the World," *livescience*, June 23, 2008, http://www.livescience.com/7509-smallpox-changed-world.html.
25. Jared Diamond, "Episode One: Out of Eden—Transcript," *Guns, Germs and Steel*, http://www.pbs.org/gunsgermssteel/show/transcript1.html.
26. C. P. Gross and K. A. Sepkowitz, "The Myth of the Medical Breakthrough: Smallpox, Vaccination, and Jenner Reconsidered," *International Journal of Infectious Diseases*, July 1998, https://www.researchgate.net/publication/13454451_Gross_CP_Sepkowitz_KAThe_myth_of_the_medical_breakthrough_smallpox_vaccination_and_Jenner_reconsidered_Int_J_Infect_Dis_354-60.
27. Richard Gordon, *The Alarming History of Medicine* (New York: St. Martin's Griffin, 1993), p. 101.
28. Cook, *Born to Die*, p. 67.
29. David M. Turner and Kevin Stagg, *Social Histories of Disability and Deformity: Bodies, Images and Experiences* (Abingdon, UK: Routledge, 2006), p. 52.
30. John Bell, *Bell's British Theatre, Consisting of the Most Esteemed English Plays*, Vol. 17 (1780), Google digital from the library of Harvard University, https://archive.org/details/bellsbritishthe19bellgoog, p. 33.

31. Lady Mary Wortley Montagu, "Lady Mary Wortley Montagu on Small Pox in Turkey [Letter]," annotated by Lynda Payne, *Children and Youth in History*, Item #157, https://chnm.gmu.edu/cyh/primary-sources/157.

32. Ibid.

33. William Osler, "Man's Redemption of Man," *American Magazine*, April 1911 to November 2010, digitized by Google, https://books.google.com/books?id=I-EvAAAAMAAJ&pg=PA251&lpg=PA251&dq=Here+I+would+like+to+say+a+word+or+two+upon+one+of+the+most+terrible+of+all+acute+infections,+the+one+of+which+we+first+learned+the+control+through+the+work+of+Jenner.+A+great+deal+of+literature+has+been+distributed&source=bl&ots=ijHGbb6zsT&sig=FbS0JbRnrwol-CKqaOtdRLKxSYeg&hl=en&sa=X&ved=0ahUKEwjoqqHooavMAhWHtYMKHU6yB3UQ6AEIHTAA#v=onepage&q=Here%20I%20would%20like%20to%20say%20a%20word%20or%20two%20upon%20one%20of%20the%20most%20terrible%20of%20all%20acute%20infec tions%2C%20the%20one%20of%20which%20we%20first%20learned%20the%20control%20through%20the%20work%20of%20Jen ner.%20A%20great%20deal%20of%20literature%20has%20been%20dis tributed&f=false.

34. Brian Deer, "MMR Doctor Given Legal Aid Thousands," *Sunday Times*, December 31, 2006, http://briandeer.com/mmr/st-dec-2006.htm.

35. Brian Deer, "Exposed: Andrew Wakefield and the MMR-Autism Fraud," briandeer.com, http://briandeer.com/mmr/lancet-summary.htm.

36. Sarah Boseley, "Lancet Retracts 'Utterly False' MMR Paper," *Guardian*, February 2, 2010, http://www.theguardian.com/society/2010/feb/02/lan cet-retracts-mmr-paper.

37. "Measles," Media Center—Fact Sheet, World Health Organization, March 2016, http://www.who.int/mediacentre/factsheets/fs286/en/.

Syphilis

1. Monica-Maria Stapelberg, *Through the Darkness: Glimpses into the History of Western Medicine* (UK: Crux, 2016), p. 74.

2. Abraham Hertz and Emanuel Lincoln, *The Hidden Lincoln: From the Letters and Papers of William H. Herndon* (New York: Viking Press, 1938), p. 259.

3. Philip Weiss, "Beethoven's Hair Tells All!," *New York Times Magazine*, November 29, 1998, http://www.nytimes.com/1998/11/29/magazine/beethoven-s-hair-tells-all.html?pagewanted=all.

4. "Diseases and Conditions: Syphilis," Mayo Clinic, January 2, 2014, http://www.mayoclinic.org/diseases-conditions/syphilis/basics/sym ptoms/con-20021862.

5. Deborah Hayden, *Pox: Genius, Madness and the Mysteries of Syphilis* (New York: Basic Books, 2003), p. 179.

6. C. G. Jung, *Nietzsche's Zarathustra: Notes of the Seminar Given in 1934–*

1939, 2 vols., edited by James L. Jarrett (Princeton: Princeton University Press, 2012), e-book, location 609.

7. Hayden, *Pox*, p. 177.
8. Walter Stewart, *Nietzsche: My Sister and I: A Critical Study* (Bloomington, IN: Xlibris, 2007), p. 91.
9. Hayden, *Pox*, p. 177.
10. Ibid., p. 178.
11. Ibid., p. 151.
12. Upton Sinclair, *Damaged Goods* (Philadelphia: John C. Winston, 1913), p. 67.
13. Vickram Chahal, "The Evolution of Nasal Reconstruction: The Origins of Plastic Surgery," Proceedings of the 10th Annual History of Medicine Days, University of Calgary, Calgary, Alberta, March 23–24, 2001, http://www.ucalgary.ca/uofc/Others/HOM/Dayspapers2001.pdf.
14. Stapelberg, *Through the Darkness*, p. 178.
15. William Eamon, *The Professor of Secrets: Mystery, Medicine, and Alchemy in Renaissance Italy* (Washington: National Geographic Society, 2010), p. 96.
16. Ibid.
17. John Frith, "Syphilis—Its Early History and Treatment until Penicillin and the Debate on Its Origins," *Journal of Military and Veterans' Health*, Nov. 2012, http://jmvh.org/article/syphilis-its-early-history-and-treatment-until-penicillin-and-the-debate-on-its-origins/.
18. Lois N. Magner, *A History of Medicine* (New York: Marcel Dekker, 1992), p. 191.
19. Lawrence I. Conrad, Michael Neve, Vivian Nutton, Roy Porter, and Andrew Wear, *The Western Medical Tradition: 800 BC to AD 1800* (Cambridge: Cambridge University Press, 1995), p. 308.
20. Kayla Jo Blackmon, "Public Power, Private Matters: The American Social Hygiene Association and the Policing of Sexual Health in the Progressive Era," thesis, University of Montana, Missoula, MT, May 2014, p. 30, http://etd.lib.umt.edu/theses/available/etd-06262014-081201/unrestricted/publicpowerprivatemattersblackmanthesisupload.pdf.
21. Angela Serratore, "Lady Colin: The Victorian Not-Quite-Divorcee Who Scandalized London," Jezebel.com, November 11, 2014, http://jezebel.com/lady-colin-the-victorian-not-quite-divorcee-who-scanda-1650034397.
22. Anne Jordan, *Love Well the Hour: The Life of Lady Colin Campbell (1857–1911)* (Leicester: Matador, 2010), p. 92.
23. Serratore, "Lady Colin."
24. *Blackwood's Edinburgh Magazine*, April 1818 (Ann Arbor: University of Michigan Library, 2009), p. 554. https://books.google.com/books?id=res7AQAAMAAJ&pg=PA554&lpg=PA554&dq=No+Nose+club+edinburgh+magazine&source=bl&ots=W4wo-3O32h&sig

=uIMQaVaBbfUR2jhEGvRsl_GWZZ4&hl=en&sa=X&ved=0ahUKEwij
zYSmx57MAhVG3mMKHRQ9AkEQ6AEIMjAD#v=onepage&q
=No%20Nose%20club%20edinburgh%20magazine&f=false.
25. Ibid., p. 555.
26. Ibid.

Tuberculosis

1. "What Is Tuberculosis?" National Institute of Allergy and Infectious
Diseases, March 6, 2009, http://www.niaid.nih.gov/topics/tuberculosis
/understanding/whatistb/Pages/default.aspx.
2. Henrietta Elizabeth Marshall, *Uncle Tom's Cabin Told to the Children*,
from the Told to the Children series, edited by Louey Chisholm (New
York: Dutton, 1904), http://utc.iath.virginia.edu/childrn/cbjackhp.html,
p. 84.
3. Edgar Allan Poe, *Great Short Works of Edgar Allan Poe*, edited by G. R.
Thompson (New York: Harper Collins, 1970), p. 95.
4. Victor Hugo, *The Works of Victor Hugo, One Volume Edition* (New York:
Collier, 1928), p. 270.
5. Helen Bynum, *Spitting Blood: The History of Tuberculosis* (Oxford:
Oxford University Press, 2012), p. 93.
6. René Dubos and Jean Dubos, *The White Plague: Tuberculosis, Man and
Society* (Boston: Little, Brown, 1996), p. 22.
7. John Cordy Jeaffreson, *The Real Lord Byron: New Views of the Poet's Life*,
Vol. 2 (1883; reprint, Ann Arbor: University of Michigan Library, Hard
press, 2012), p. 259.
8. Dubos and Dubos, *The White Plague*, p. 9.
9. James Clark, *Medical Notes on Climate, Diseases, Hospitals, and Medical
Schools, in France, Italy and Switzerland* (1820; reprint, Cambridge:
Cambridge University Press, 2013), p. 94.
10. Nicholas Roe, *John Keats: A New Life* (New Haven, CT: Yale University
Press, 2012), p. 389.
11. Daniel H. Whitney, *The Family Physician, and Guide to Health, Together
with the History, Causes, Symptoms and Treatment of the Asiatic Cholera,
a Glossary Explaining the Most Difficult Words That Occur in Medical
Science, and a Copious Index, to Which Is Added an Appendix* (1833),
U.S. National Library of Medicine site, https://archive.org/details/2577
008R.nlm.nih.gov, p. 62.
12. Clark Lawlor, *Consumption and Literature: The Making of the Romantic
Disease* (New York: Palgrave Macmillan, 2007), p. 45.
13. John Keats, *The Letters of John Keats: Volume 2*, edited by Hyder Edward
Rollins (Cambridge, MA: Harvard University Press, 1958), p. 364.
14. Lawlor, *Consumption and Literature*, p. 17.
15. Ibid.
16. Whitney, *The Family Physician*, p. 60.

17. Lawlor, *Consumption and Literature*, p. 157.
18. Ibid., p. 50.
19. John Frith, "History of Tuberculosis: Part 1—Phthisis, Consumption and the White Plague," *Journal of Military and Veterans' Health*, http://jmvh.org/article/history-of-tuberculosis-part-1-phthisis-consumption-and-the-white-plague/.
20. Lawlor, *Consumption and Literature*, p. 21.
21. Ibid., p. 50.
22. Ibid., p. 153.
23. Dubos and Dubos, *The White Plague*, p. 52.
24. Ibid., p. 9.
25. Bynum, *Spitting Blood*, p. 112.
26. Dubos and Dubos, *The White Plague*, p. 7.
27. Bynum, *Spitting Blood*, p. 111.
28. Dubos and Dubos, *The White Plague*, p. 17.
29. Ibid., p. 18.
30. Ibid., p. 24.
31. Lawlor, *Consumption and Literature*, p. 43.
32. Katherine Byrne, *Tuberculosis and the Victorian Literary Imagination* (Cambridge: Cambridge University Press, 2011), p. 100.
33. Lucinda Hawksley, *Lizzie Siddal: The Tragedy of a Pre-Raphaelite Supermodel* (New York: Walker, 2004), p. 985.
34. Byrne, *Tuberculosis*, p. 100.
35. Ibid., p. 101.
36. Leo Tolstoy, *Anna Karenina*, Christian Classics Ethereal Library. Read online at http://www.ccel.org/ccel/tolstoy/karenina, section vi, p. xvii.
37. Byrne, *Tuberculosis*, p. 101.
38. Lawlor, *Consumption and Literature*, p. 188.
39. Ibid., p. 198.
40. "Tuberculosis," Centers for Disease Control and Prevention, December 9, 2011, http://www.cdc.gov/tb/topic/treatment/.
41. "International Drug Price Indicator Guide—Vaccine, Bcg," Management Sciences for Health, 2014, http://erc.msh.org/dmpguide/resultsdetail.cfm?language=english&code=BCG00A&s_year=2014&year=2014&str=&desc=Vaccine%2C%20BCG&pack=new&frm=POWDER&rte=INJ&class_code2=19%2E3%2E&supplement=&class_name=%2819%2E3%2E%29 Vaccines%3Cbr%3E.

Cholera

1. Stephen Halliday, "Death and Miasma in Victorian London: An Obstinate Belief," *British Medical Journal*, October 23, 2001, http://www.bmj.com/content/323/7327/1469.
2. Ibid.

3. Ibid.
4. Ibid.
5. Steven Johnson, *The Ghost Map: The Story of London's Most Terrifying Epidemic—and How It Changed Science, Cities, and the Modern World* (New York: Penguin, 2006), p. 29.
6. Steven Johnson, "How the 'Ghost Map' Helped End a Killer Disease," TEDsalon, November 2006, https://www.ted.com/talks/steven_johnson _tours_the_ghost_map?language=en#t-59501.
7. Charles Dickens, "The Troubled Water Question," *Household Words, a Weekly Journal*, April 13, 1850, https://books.google.com/books?id =MPNAAQAAMAAJ&pg=PA53&lpg=PA53&dq=charles+dickens +troubled+water+question&source=bl&ots=aVNLBwQOCh&sig =oAGlhCUH9fzUJik8llHyOxoCjSI&hl=en&sa=X&ved=0ahUKEwiho5u K8OHLAhWBbiYKHV5iChkQ6AEILTAD#v=onepage&q=charles%20 dickens%20troubled%20water%20question&f=false.
8. Stephen Halliday, *The Great Stink of London: Sir Joseph Bazalgette and the Cleansing of the Victorian Metropolis* (Gloucestershire: History Press, 2001), p. 39.
9. Johnson, *The Ghost Map*, Kindle location 3539.
10. John Snow, "John Snow's Teetotal Address," Spring 1836, from the *British Temperance Advocate*, 1888, UCLA Department of Epidemiology, School of Public Health, http://www.ph.ucla.edu/epi/snow/teetotal.html.
11. Ibid.
12. Kathleen Tuthill, "John Snow and the Broad Street Pump," *Cricket*, November 2003, UCLA Department of Epidemiology, School of Public Health, http://www.ph.ucla.edu/epi/snow/snowcricketarticle.html.
13. John Snow, "On Chloroform and Other Anaesthetics: Their Action and Administration," 1858, Wood Library Museum, http://www.woodlibrary-museum.org/ebooks/item/643/snow,-john.-on-chloroform-and-other -anaesthetics,-their-action-and-administration-(with-a-memoir-of-the -author,-by-benjamin-w.-richardson).
14. Johnson, *The Ghost Map*, Kindle location 59.
15. Sandra Hempel, "John Snow," *Lancet* 381, no. 9874 (April 13, 2013), http:// www.thelancet.com/journals/lancet/article/PIIS0140-6736(13)60830-2 /fulltext?elsca1=TW.
16. Danny Dorling, *Unequal Health: The Scandal of Our Times* (Bristol: Policy Press, 2013).
17. Johnson, *The Ghost Map*, Kindle location 70.
18. John Snow, "On the Mode of Communication of Cholera," pamphlet (1849), reviewed in the *London Medical Gazette*, September 14, 1849, John Snow Archive and Research Companion, http://johnsnow.matrix.msu .edu/work.php?id=15-78-28.
19. Ibid.

20. Johnson, *The Ghost Map*, Kindle location 56.
21. Tuthill, "John Snow."
22. Peter Vinten-Johansen Howard Brody, Nigel Paneth, Stephen Rachman, and Michael Rip, *Cholera, Chloroform, and the Science of Medicine: A Life of John Snow* (Oxford: Oxford University Press, 2003).
23. "Reverend Henry Whitehead," UCLA Department of Epidemiology, School of Public Health, http://www.ph.ucla.edu/epi/snow/whitehead.html.
24. Johnson, *The Ghost Map*, Kindle edition, location 148.
25. "Snow's Testimony," UCLA Department of Epidemiology, School of Public Health, http://www.ph.ucla.edu/epi/snow/snows_testimony.html.
26. Reuters. "Why Bad Smells Make You Gag," ABC Science, March 5, 2008, http://www.abc.net.au/science/articles/2008/03/05/2180489.htm.
27. "Snow's Testimony."
28. Ibid.
29. Johnson, *The Ghost Map*, Kindle location 183.
30. John Snow, "Letter to the Right Honourable Sir Benjamin Hall, Bart., President of the General Board of Health," July 12, 1855, original pamphlet courtesy of the Historical Library, Yale University Medical School, the John Snow Archive and Research Companion, http://johnsnow.matrix.msu.edu/work.php?id=15-78-5A.
31. Dorling, *Unequal Health*, p. 24.
32. "Reverend Henry Whitehead."
33. Ibid.
34. Ibid.
35. Hempel, "John Snow."
36. Vinten-Johansen et al., *Cholera, Chloroform, and the Science of Medicine*, p. 395.
37. Hempel, "John Snow."
38. "Retrospect of Cholera in the East of London," *Lancet* 2 (September 29, 1866), https://books.google.com/books?id=SxxAAAAAcAAJ&pg=PA1317&lpg=PA1317&dq=The+Lancet+london+Cholera+in+the+east+of+london++September+29+1866&source=bl&ots=Z-bAnpDI5s&sig=ZgLRBf3WznA2gzwsbgZAzmuQBlE&hl=en&sa=X&ved=0ahUKEwimtf-Ik-LLAhUDKCYKHQQ5DwUQ6AEIHDAA#v=onepage&q=The%20Lancet%20london%20Cholera%20in%20the%20east%20of%20london%20%20September%2029%201866&f=false.
39. Ibid.
40. Snow, "On Chloroform and Other Anaesthetics."

Leprosy

1. "St. Damien of Molokai," Catholic Online, http://www.catholic.org/saints/saint.php?saint_id=2817.
2. Stephen Brown, "Pope Canonizes Leper Saint Damien, Hailed by Obama,"

edited by David Stamp, Reuters, October 11, 2009, http://www.reuters
.com/article/2009/10/11/us-pope-saints-idUSTRE59A0YW20091011.

3. "St. Damien of Molokai."

4. King James Bible (New York: American Bible Society, 1999; New York: Bartleby.com, 2000).

5. Kate Yandell, "The Leprosy Bacillus, circa 1873," *TheScientist*, October 1, 2013, http://www.the-scientist.com/?articles.view/articleNo/37619/title /The-Leprosy-Bacillus—circa-1873/.

6. K. Blom, "Armauer Hansen and Human Leprosy Transmission: Medical Ethics and Legal Rights," 1973, U.S. National Library of Medicine, http://www.ncbi.nlm.nih.gov/pubmed/4592244.

7. "An Act to Prevent the Spread of Leprosy, 1865," January 1865, National Park Service, http://www.nps.gov/kala/learn/historyculture/1865.htm.

8. Jack London, *Tales of the Pacific* (London: Penguin, 1989), p. 173.

9. Joseph Dutton, "Molokai," *The Catholic Encyclopedia: An International Work of Reference on the Constitution, Doctrine, Discipline, and History of the Catholic Church*, vol. 10 (New York: Encyclopedia Press, January 1, 1913), p. 445.

10. Richard Stewart, *Leper Priest of Molokai: The Father Damien Story* (Honolulu: University of Hawaii Press, 2000), p. 81.

11. "Damien the Leper," Franciscans of St. Anthony's Guild, 1974, Eternal World Television Network, https://www.ewtn.com/library/MARY/DAM IEN.HTM. (Originally published in 1974 by the Franciscans of St. Anthony's Guild, Patterson, New Jersey.)

12. Gavan Daws, *Holy Man: Father Damien of Molokai* (Honolulu: University of Hawaii Press, 1989), p. 113.

13. "Appendix M: Special Report from Rev. J. Damien, Catholic Priest at Kalawao, March 1886," Report of the Board of Health, https://books .google.com/books?id=C7JNAAAAMAAJ&pg=PR110&lpg=PR110&dq =Special+report+J.+Damien+1886&source=bl&ots=R1-cZ_SXPp&sig =M1DwLciA7V1IR-D-fKmCsPaen7I&hl=en&sa=X&ved=0ahUKEwj0 -fvLsuLLAhWBLyYKHdSjArUQ6AEIKDAE#v=onepage&q=Special %20report%20J.%20Damien%201886&f=false.

14. Daws, *Holy Man*, p. 73.

15. Stewart, *Leper Priest of Molokai*, p. 80.

16. John Farrow, *Damien the Leper: A Life of Magnificent Courage, Devotion & Spirit* (New York: Image Books [Doubleday], 1954), p. 20.

17. Stewart, *Leper Priest of Molokai*, p. 17.

18. Ibid., p. 22.

19. Jan de Volder, *The Spirit of Father Damien: The Leper Priest—a Saint for Our Time* (San Francisco: Ignatius Press, 2010), p. 3.

20. Stewart, *Leper Priest of Molokai*, p. 22.

21. Ibid., p. 23.

22. Farrow, *Damien the Leper*, p. 34.

23. Stewart, *Leper Priest of Molokai*, p. 27.
24. Ibid., p. 36.
25. Ibid., p. 86.
26. Ibid., p. 80.
27. Vincent J. O'Malley, *Saints of North America* (Huntington, IN: Our Sunday Visitor, 2004), p. 200.
28. Stewart, *Leper Priest of Molokai*, p. 90.
29. Ibid.
30. Hilde Eynikel, *Molokai: The Story of Father Damien* (St. Paul's/Alba House, 1999), p. 75.
31. Farrow, *Damien the Leper*, p. 123.
32. "Damien the Leper."
33. O'Malley, *Saints of North America*, p. 201.
34. Daws, *Holy Man*, p. 84.
35. Farrow, *Damien the Leper*, p. 123.
36. "Damien the Leper."
37. Ibid.
38. Daws, *Holy Man*, p. 116.
39. Ibid., pp. 115–16.
40. Stewart, *Leper Priest of Molokai*, p. 100.
41. Nicholas Senn, "Father Damien, the Leper Hero," *Journal of the American Medical Association*, August 27, 1904, https://books.google.com/books?pg=PA605&lpg=PA607&sig=mJi_mLzilMWH9Ac7pkeCYkwZxXg&ei=c6KySpScI9GklAe3y4H5Dg&ct=result&id=e-sBAAAAYAAJ&ots=LaTpBrjyQJ#v=onepage&q&f=false pp. 301–11.
42. Volder, *The Spirit of Father Damien*, p. 72.
43. Ibid., p. 74.
44. Daws, *Holy Man*, p. 113.
45. Ibid., p. 112.
46. Farrow, *Damien the Leper*, p. 172.
47. "Damien the Leper."
48. Farrow, *Damien the Leper*, p. 192.
49. Ibid., p. 200.
50. Ibid., p. 233.
51. Ibid., p. 237.
52. Tony Gould, *A Disease Apart: Leprosy in the Modern World* (New York: St. Martin's Press, 2005), p. 143.
53. Ibid., p. 144.
54. Ibid., p. 198.
55. Volder, *The Spirit of Father Damien*, p. 198.

Typhoid

1. Susan Campbell Bartoletti, *Terrible Typhoid Mary: A True Story of the Deadliest Cook in America* (New York: Houghton Mifflin Harcourt, 2015), p. 15.

2. Dr. Annie Gray, "How to Make Ice Cream the Victorian Way," English Heritage website, http://www.english-heritage.org.uk/visit/pick-of-season/how-to-make-victorian-ice-cream/.
3. Bartoletti, *Terrible Typhoid Mary*, p. 23.
4. Donald G. McNeil Jr., "Bacteria Study Offers Clues to Typhoid Mary Mystery," *New York Times*, August 26, 2013, http://www.nytimes.com/2013/08/27/health/bacteria-study-offers-clues-to-typhoid-mary-mystery.html?_r=0.
5. Mary Lowth, "Typhoid and Paratyphoid Fever," Patient website, February 25, 2015, http://patient.info/doctor/typhoid-and-paratyphoid-fever-pro.
6. Bartoletti, *Terrible Typhoid Mary*, p. 43.
7. George A. Soper, "The Work of a Chronic Typhoid Germ Distributor," 1907, Primary Sources: Workshops in American History, https://www.learner.org/workshops/primarysources/disease/docs/soper2.html.
8. Ibid.
9. Ibid.
10. Judith Walzer Leavitt, *Typhoid Mary: Captive to the Public's Health* (Boston: Beacon Press, 1996), pp. 40–41.
11. Soper, "The Work of a Chronic Typhoid Germ Distributor."
12. Antonia Petrash, *More Than Petticoats: Remarkable New York Women* (TwoDot, 2001), p. 121.
13. S. Josephine Baker, *Fighting for Life* (1939; reprint, New York: New York Times Review of Books, 2013), p. 73.
14. Ibid., p. 75.
15. Leavitt, *Typhoid Mary*, p. 9.
16. Petrash, *More Than Petticoats*, p. 118.
17. Bartoletti, *Terrible Typhoid Mary*, p. 84.
18. Soper, "The Work of a Chronic Typhoid Germ Distributor."
19. "Typhoid Mary Wants Liberty," *Richmond Planet*, July 10, 1909, Chronicling America: Historic American Newspapers, Library of Congress, http://chroniclingamerica.loc.gov/lccn/sn84025841/1909-07-10/ed-1/seq-7/#date1=1836&sort=relevance&rows=20&words=MARY+TYPHOID&searchType=basic&sequence=0&index=0&state=&date2=1922&proxtext=typhoid+mary&y=0&x=0&dateFilterType=yearRange&page=2.
20. Leavitt, *Typhoid Mary*, p. 94.
21. Ibid., p. 32.
22. Mary Mallon, "In Her Own Words," NOVA, http://www.pbs.org/wgbh/nova/typhoid/letter.html.
23. Baker, *Fighting for Life*, p. 76.
24. Leavitt, *Typhoid Mary*, p. 128.
25. Bartoletti, *Terrible Typhoid Mary*, p. 108.
26. Mallon, "In Her Own Words."
27. Ibid.

28. Ibid.
29. Leavitt, *Typhoid Mary*, p. 56.
30. William H. Park, "Typhoid Bacilli Carriers," 1908, Primary Sources: Workshops in American History, https://www.learner.org/workshops /primarysources/disease/docs/park2.html.
31. Ibid.
32. Bartoletti, *Terrible Typhoid Mary*, p. 119.
33. Leavitt, *Typhoid Mary*, p. 104.
34. Ibid., p. 55.
35. Ibid., p. 117.
36. Ibid., p. 87.
37. Bartoletti, *Terrible Typhoid Mary*, p. 121.
38. Baker, *Fighting for Life*, p. 76.
39. Leavitt, *Typhoid Mary*, p. 135.
40. John B. Huber, "'Microbe Carriers'—the Newly Discovered," *Richmond Times-Dispatch*, July 11, 1915, Chronicling America: Historic American Newspapers, Library of Congress, http://chroniclingamerica.loc.gov/lccn /sn83045389/1915-07-11/ed-1/seq-42/#date1=1915&index=0&rows=20 &words=typhoid+Typhoid&searchType=basic&sequence=0&state= &date2=1915&proxtext=typhoid&y=0&x=0&dateFilterType=yearRange &page=1.
41. Ibid.
42. Ibid.
43. Bartoletti, *Terrible Typhoid Mary*, p. 43.
44. "Mystery of the Poison Guest at Wealthy Mrs. Case's Party," *Richmond Times-Dispatch*, August 22, 1920, Chronicling America: Historic American Newspapers, Library of Congress, http://chroniclingamerica.loc.gov /lccn/sn83045389/1920-08-22/ed-1/seq-51/#date1=1907&index=3&rows =20&words=Mary+Typhoid+typhoid&searchType=basic&sequence=0 &state=&date2=1922&proxtext=typhoid+mary+&y=12&x=1&dateFil terType=yearRange&page=1.
45. Bartoletti, *Terrible Typhoid Mary*, p. 150.
46. Baker, *Fighting for Life*, p. 76.

Spanish Flu

1. John M. Barry, *The Great Influenza: The Story of the Deadliest Pandemic in History* (New York: Penguin, 2004), pp. 104–8.
2. Alfred W. Crosby, *America's Forgotten Pandemic: The Influenza of 1918* (Cambridge: Cambridge University Press, 2003), Kindle location, p. 452.
3. Barry, *The Great Influenza*, p. 239.
4. "Influenza 1918," a complete transcript of the program, *American Experience*, PBS.org, http://www.pbs.org/wgbh/americanexperience/features /transcript/influenza-transcript/.
5. Barry, *The Great Influenza*, p. 109.

6. Ibid., p. 109.
7. Ibid., p. 110.
8. Jeffrey Greene and Karen Moline, *The Bird Flu Pandemic: Can It Happen? Will It Happen? How to Protect Your Family If It Does* (New York: St. Martin's Press, 2006), p. 41.
9. Board of Global Health, Institute of Medicine of the National Academies, "The Threat of Pandemic Influenza: Are We Ready?" workshop overview, National Center for Biotechnology Information, 2005, http://www.ncbi.nlm.nih.gov/books/NBK22148/.
10. Roy Greenslade, "First World War: How State and Press Kept Truth off the Front Page," *Guardian*, July 27, 2014, http://www.theguardian.com/media/2014/jul/27/first-world-war-state-press-reporting.
11. Barry, *The Great Influenza*, p. 140.
12. "Influenza 1918."
13. Antoni Trilla, Guillem Trilla, and Carolyn Daer, "The 1918 'Spanish Flu' in Spain," *Oxford Journals, Clinical Infectious Diseases* 47, no. 5 (2008), http://cid.oxfordjournals.org/content/47/5/668.full.
14. Barry, *The Great Influenza*, p. 170.
15. Crosby, *America's Forgotten Pandemic*, p. 27.
16. Trilla et al., "The 1918 'Spanish Flu' in Spain."
17. Juliet Nicholson, "The War Was Over but Spanish Flu Would Kill Millions More," *Telegraph*, November 11, 2009, http://www.telegraph.co.uk/news/health/6542203/The-war-was-over-but-Spanish-Flu-would-kill-millions-more.html#disqus_thread.
18. Crosby, *America's Forgotten Pandemic*, p. 34.
19. Barry, *The Great Influenza*, p. 168.
20. "Influenza 1918."
21. Christine M. Kreiser, "1918 Spanish Influenza Outbreak: The Enemy Within," HistoryNet website, October 27, 2006, http://www.historynet.com/1918-spanish-influenza-outbreak-the-enemy-within.htm.
22. "Influenza 1918."
23. Randy Dotinga, "5 Surprising Facts about Woodrow Wilson and Racism," *Christian Science Monitor*, December 14, 2013, http://www.csmonitor.com/Books/chapter-and-verse/2015/1214/5-surprising-facts-about-Woodrow-Wilson-and-racism.
24. Randy Barnett, "The Volokh Conspiracy: Expunging Woodrow Wilson from Official Places of Honor," *Washington Post*, June 25, 2015, https://www.washingtonpost.com/news/volokh-conspiracy/wp/2015/06/25/expunging-woodrow-wilson-from-official-places-of-honor/.
25. "Woodrow Wilson," *The Great Pandemic—The United States in 1918–1919*, United States Department of Health and Human Services, http://www.flu.gov/pandemic/history/1918/biographies/wilson/.
26. "Over There," a song by George M. Cohan, Wikipedia, https://en.wikipedia.org/wiki/Over_There.

27. "Influenza 1918."
28. Crosby, *America's Forgotten Pandemic*, p. 35.
29. "Influenza 1918."
30. Tom Ewing, "Influenza in the News: Using Newspapers to Understand a Public Health Crisis," National Digital Newspaper—Program Awardee Conference, September 26, 2012, http://www.flu1918.lib.vt.edu/wp-content /uploads/2012/11/NDNP_Ewing_Influenza_25Sept2012.pdf.
31. Barry, *The Great Influenza*, p. 209.
32. Ibid., p. 215.
33. Kreiser, "1918 Spanish Influenza Outbreak."
34. "The Flu of 1918," *Pennsylvania Gazette*, October 28, 1998, http://www .upenn.edu/gazette/1198/lynch2.html.
35. Ibid.
36. Greene and Moline, *The Bird Flu Pandemic*, p. 23.
37. Katherine Anne Porter, *Pale Horse, Pale Rider: Three Short Novels* (New York: Harcourt Brace & Company, 1939; reprinted 1990), p. 158.
38. Barry, *The Great Influenza*, p. 210.
39. "Scientific Nursing Halting Epidemic," *Philadelphia Inquirer*, October 15, 1918, from the Influenza Encyclopedia, University of Michigan Library, http://quod.lib.umich.edu/f/flu/3990flu.0007.993/1.
40. Barry, *The Great Influenza*, p. 239.
41. Charles Hardy, "'Please Let Me Put Him in a Macaroni Box'—the Spanish Influenza of 1918 in Philadelphia," WHYY-FM radio program *The Influenza Pandemic of 1918*, Philadelphia, 1984, History Matters, http:// historymatters.gmu.edu/d/13/.
42. Barry, *The Great Influenza*, p. 333.
43. "Influenza 1918."
44. Ibid.
45. "The Great Pandemic—New York," United States Department of Health and Human Services, http://www.flu.gov/pandemic/history/1918/your _state/northeast/newyork/.
46. Ibid.
47. Barry, *The Great Influenza*, p. 340.
48. "Influenza 1918."
49. Barry, *The Great Influenza*, p. 252.
50. Ibid., p. 251.
51. Ewing, "Influenza in the News: Using Newspapers to Understand a Public Health Crisis."
52. Barry, *The Great Influenza*, p. 189.
53. Greene and Moline, *The Bird Flu Pandemic*, p. 40.
54. Nicholson, "The War Was Over."
55. "The Flu of 1918."
56. Nicholson, "The War Was Over."
57. "The Flu of 1918."

58. Nicholson, "The War Was Over."
59. Barry, *The Great Influenza*, p. 228.
60. Nicholson, "The War Was Over."
61. "Influenza 1918."
62. Nicholson, "The War Was Over."
63. Board of Global Health, Institute of Medicine of the National Academies, *The Threat of Pandemic Influenza: Are We Ready?* workshop summary edited by Stacey L. Knobler, Alison Mack, Adel Mahmoud, and Stanley M. Lemon (Washington: National Academies Press, 2005), http://www.ncbi.nlm.nih.gov/books/NBK22156/.
64. "The Great Pandemic—New York."
65. Barry, *The Great Influenza*, p. 338.
66. "Influenza 1918."
67. James T. Willerson, "The Great Enemy—Infectious Disease," edited by S. Ward Casscells and Mohammad Madjid, Texas Heart Institute Journal, 2004, http://www.ncbi.nlm.nih.gov/pmc/articles/PMC387424/.
68. Steve Connor, "American Scientists Controversially Recreate Deadly Spanish Flu," *Independent*, June 11, 2014, http://www.independent.co.uk/news/science/american-scientists-controversially-recreate-deadly-spanish-flu-virus-9529707.html.
69. Barry, *The Great Influenza*, p. 469.

Encephalitis Lethargica
1. Joel A. Vilensky, "Sleeping Princes and Princesses: The Encephalitis Lethargica Epidemic of the 1920s and a Contemporary Evaluation of the Disease," presentation slides, 2008, http://slideplayer.com/slide/3899891/.
2. Joel A. Vilensky, *Encephalitis Lethargica: During and After the Epidemic* (Oxford: Oxford University Press, 2011), Kindle edition, location 336.
3. Molly Caldwell Crosby, *Asleep: The Forgotten Epidemic That Remains One of Medicine's Greatest Mysteries* (New York: Berkley Books, 2010), Kindle edition, location 7.
4. Ibid.
5. Vilensky, *Encephalitis Lethargica*, Kindle location 368.
6. Crosby, *Asleep*, Kindle location 6.
7. Vilensky, *Encephalitis Lethargica*, Kindle location 563–64.
8. Ibid., Kindle location 368.
9. Crosby, *Asleep*, Kindle location 94.
10. Ibid., Kindle location 85.
11. Oliver Sacks, *Awakenings* (New York: Vintage Books, 1999), p. 18.
12. Ibid., p. 111.
13. Gina Kolata, *The Story of the Great Influenza Pandemic of 1918 and the Search for the Virus That Caused It* (New York: Touchstone, 1999), p. 344.
14. Crosby, *Asleep*, Kindle location 13.

15. Vilensky, *Encephalitis Lethargica*, Kindle location 3815.
16. Crosby, *Asleep*, Kindle location 9.
17. Vilensky, *Encephalitis Lethargica*, Kindle location 550.
18. Ann H. Reid, Sherman McCall, James M. Henry, and Jeffrey K. Taubenberger, "Experimenting on the Past: The Enigma of von Economo's Encephalitis Lethargica," *Journal of Neuropathology and Experimental Neurology*, July 2001, http://jnen.oxfordjournals.org/content/60/7/663.
19. Vilensky, *Encephalitis Lethargica*, Kindle location 3839–42.
20. Crosby, *Asleep*, Kindle location 11.
21. Vilensky, *Encephalitis Lethargica*, Kindle location 582–83.
22. Crosby, *Asleep*, Kindle location 13.
23. Ibid., Kindle location 60.
24. Vilensky, *Encephalitis Lethargica*, Kindle location 3911–13.
25. Crosby, *Asleep*, Kindle location 140.
26. Ibid., Kindle location 15.
27. Sacks, *Awakenings*, p. 18.
28. Crosby, *Asleep*, Kindle location 145.
29. Sacks, *Awakenings*, p. 62.
30. Ibid., p. 44.
31. Ibid., pp. 40, 44, 62.
32. Ibid., p. 129.
33. Ibid.
34. Sue Carswell, "Oliver Sacks," *People*, February 11, 1991, http://www.people.com/people/archive/article/0,20114432,00.html.
35. Ibid.
36. "Parkinson Disease," *New York Times Health Guide*, September 16, 2013, http://www.nytimes.com/health/guides/disease/parkinsons-disease/levadopa-(l-dopa).html.
37. Sacks, *Awakenings*, p. 80.
38. Carswell, "Oliver Sacks."
39. Sacks, *Awakenings*, p. 31.

Lobotomies

1. Howard Dully and Charles Fleming, *My Lobotomy* (New York: Three Rivers Press, 2008), p. 78.
2. "Introduction: The Lobotomist," *American Experience*, PBS, http://www.pbs.org/wgbh/americanexperience/features/introduction/lobotomist-introduction/.
3. John M. Harlow, "Recovery from the Passage of an Iron Bar Through the Head," Publications of the Massachusetts Medical Society, 1868, Wikisource, https://en.wikisource.org/wiki/Recovery_from_the_passage_of_an_iron_bar_through_the_head.
4. Jack El-Hai, *The Lobotomist: A Maverick Medical Genius and His Tragic*

Quest to Rid the World of Mental Illness (Hoboken: Wiley, 2005), Kindle edition, location 116.

5. Kate Clifford Larson, *Rosemary: The Hidden Kennedy Daughter* (New York: Houghton Mifflin Harcourt, 2015), p. 172.

6. John B. Dynes and James L. Poppen, "Lobotomy for Intractable Pain," *Journal of the American Medical Association* 140, no. 1 (May 7, 1949), http://jama.jamanetwork.com/article.aspx?articleid=304291.

7. Larson, *Rosemary,* p. 180.

8. Ibid.

9. Glenn Frankel, "D.C. Neurosurgeon Pioneered 'Operation Icepick' Technique," *Washington Post,* April 7, 1980.

10. Dully and Fleming, *My Lobotomy,* p. 85.

11. "My Lobotomy," *All Things Considered,* SoundPortraits Productions, November 16, 2005, http://soundportraits.org/on-air/my_lobotomy/transcript.php.

12. Dynes and Poppen, "Lobotomy for Intractable Pain."

13. Ibid.

14. Ward Harkavy, "The Scary Days When Thousands Were Lobotomized on Long Island," *Village Voice,* October 26, 1999, http://www.villagevoice.com/long-island-voice/the-scary-days-when-thousands-were-lobotomized-on-long-island-7155435.

15. Ibid.

16. "Moniz Develops Lobotomy for Mental Illness, 1935," People and Discoveries, ETV Education, 1998, PBS.org, http://www.pbs.org/wgbh/aso/databank/entries/dh35lo.html.

17. Frank T. Vertosick Jr., "Lobotomy's Back," *Discover,* October 1997, http://discovermagazine.com/1997/oct/lobotomysback1240.

18. Eric Weiner, "Nobel Panel Urged to Rescind Prize for Lobotomies," NPR.org., August 10, 2005, http://www.npr.org/templates/story/story.php?storyId=4794007.

19. Mical Raz, *Lobotomy Letters: The Making of American Psychosurgery,* edited by Theodore M. Brown, Rochester Studies in Medical History series (Rochester: University of Rochester Press, 2015), p. 113.

20. Ibid., p. 113.

21. Dynes and Poppen, "Lobotomy for Intractable Pain."

22. "Introduction: The Lobotomist."

23. Dully and Fleming, *My Lobotomy,* p. 85.

24. El-Hai, *The Lobotomist,* Kindle location 3363–64.

25. Piya Kochar and Dave Isay, "My Lobotomy: Howard Dully's Story," edited by Gary Corvino, Sound Portraits Productions, NPR.org, November 16, 2005, http://www.npr.org/2005/11/16/5014080/my-lobotomy-howard-dullys-journey.

26. Dully and Fleming, *My Lobotomy,* p. 86.

27. Ibid., p. 85.
28. Hugh Levinson, "The Strange and Curious History of Lobotomy," *Magazine, BBC News*, November 8, 2011, http://www.bbc.com/news/magazine-15629160.
29. Michael M. Phillips, "The Lobotomy File, Part Two: One Doctor's Legacy," a *Wall Street Journal* special project, 2013, http://projects.wsj.com/lobotomyfiles/?ch=two.
30. Ibid.
31. Ibid.
32. Ibid.
33. Dully and Fleming, *My Lobotomy*, p. 86.
34. Larson, *Rosemary*, p. 178.
35. Ibid., p. 180.
36. Ibid., p. 178.
37. El-Hai, *The Lobotomist*, Kindle location 1695–96.
38. Ibid., Kindle location 1582.
39. Ibid., Kindle location 3202–03.
40. Ibid., Kindle location 3206–7.
41. Kochar and Isay, "My Lobotomy."
42. El-Hai, *The Lobotomist*, Kindle location 3209–11.
43. Ibid., Kindle location 3213.
44. Phillips, "The Lobotomy File, Part Two."
45. Jack D. Pressman, *Last Resort: Psychosurgery and the Limits of Medicine*, edited by Charles Rosenberg and Colin James, Cambridge History of Medicine series (Cambridge: Cambridge University Press, 2002), p. 82.
46. Tony Long, "Nov. 12, 1935: You Should (Not) Have a Lobotomy," *WIRED*, November 12, 2010, http://www.wired.com/2010/11/1112first-lobotomy/.
47. "Moniz Develops Lobotomy for Mental Illness, 1935."
48. El-Hai, *The Lobotomist*, Kindle location 189.
49. Ibid., Kindle location 3222–23.
50. Raz, *Lobotomy Letters*, pp. 108–9.
51. Dully and Fleming, *My Lobotomy*, p. 77.
52. El-Hai, *The Lobotomist*, Kindle location 3995.
53. Kochar and Isay, "My Lobotomy."

Polio

1. David M. Oshinsky, *Polio: An American Story* (Oxford: Oxford University Press, 2005), p. 5.
2. Sheila Llanas, *Jonas Salk: Medical Innovator and Polio Vaccine Developer* (Edina, MN: ABDO, 2013), p. 8.
3. Paul A. Offit, *The Cutter Incident: How America's First Polio Vaccine Led to the Growing Vaccine Crisis* (New Haven, CT: Yale University Press, 2005), Kindle edition, location 386.
4. Oshinsky, *Polio*, p. 4.

5. "Deadly Diseases: Polio," ETV Education, PBS.org, 2005 http://www.pbs.org/wgbh/rxforsurvival/series/diseases/polio.html.
6. "Polio: What You Need to Know," myDr website, January 12, 2011, http://www.mydr.com.au/kids-teens-health/polio-what-you-need-to-know.
7. "Polio and Prevention," Global Polio Eradication Initiative, http://www.polioeradication.org/polioandprevention.aspx, pp. 4–9.
8. Oshinsky, *Polio*, p. 44.
9. Ibid., p. 46.
10. Ibid., p. 47.
11. Ibid., p. 45.
12. Daniel J. Wilson, *Living with Polio: The Epidemic and Its Survivors* (Chicago: University of Chicago Press, 2005), p. 119.
13. N. M. Nielsen, K. Rostgaard, K. Juel, D. Askgaard, and P. Aaby, "Long-term Mortality after Poliomyelitis," U.S. National Library of Medicine, May 2003, PubMed.com, http://www.ncbi.nlm.nih.gov/pubmed/12859038.
14. Wilson, *Living with Polio*, p. 120.
15. Ibid.
16. Oshinsky, *Polio*, p. 49.
17. Ibid., p. 51.
18. Ibid., p. 52.
19. Ibid., p. 188.
20. Llanas, *Jonas Salk*, p. 16.
21. Oshinsky, *Polio*, p. 101.
22. Ian Musgrave, "'Toxins' in Vaccines: A Potentially Deadly Misunderstanding," *The Conversation*, November 28, 2012, http://theconversation.com/toxins-in-vaccines-a-potentially-deadly-misunderstanding-11010.
23. Oshinsky, *Polio*, p. 228.
24. Ibid., p. 171.
25. Ibid., p. 172.
26. Thompson, "The Salk Polio Vaccine."
27. "Medicine: Closing in on Polio," *Time*, March 29, 1954, http://content.time.com/time/subscriber/article/0,33009,819686-4,00.html.
28. William Lawrence, "Sacks Polio Vaccine Proves Success; Millions Will Be Immunized Soon; City Schools Begin Shots April 25, *The New York Times*, April 13, 1955, http:timemachine.nytimes.com/timemachine/1955/04/13/issue.html.
29. Oshinsky, *Polio*, p. 211.
30. Amar Prabhu, "How Much Money Did Jonas Salk Potentially Forfeit by Not Patenting the Polio Vaccine?" *Forbes*, August 9, 2012, http://www.forbes.com/sites/quora/2012/08/09/how-much-money-did-jonas-salk-potentially-forfeit-by-not-patenting-the-polio-vaccine/#1e35e3941c2d.
31. Oshinsky, *Polio*, p. 215.
32. Ibid., p. 214.
33. Ibid., p. 216.

34. Dwight D. Eisenhower, "Citation Presented to Dr. Jonas E. Salk and Accompanying Remarks," American Presidency Project, April 22, 1955, http://www.presidency.ucsb.edu/ws/?pid=10457.

35. Ibid.

36. Stanley Plotkin, "'Herd Immunity': A Rough Guide," Oxford Journals: Clinical Infectious Diseases 52, no. 7 (2011), http://cid.oxfordjournals.org /content/52/7/911.full.

37. "Measles (MCV)—Data by Country," Global Health Observatory data repository, World Health Organization, http://apps.who.int/gho/data /node.main.A826?_ga=1.149767604.366030890.1401971125.

38. Paul A. Offit, The Cutter Incident: How America's First Polio Vaccine Led to the Growing Vaccine Crisis (New Haven, CT: Yale University Press, 2005), Kindle edition, location 178.

39. Ibid., Kindle location 2075.

40. Oshinsky, Polio, p. 255.

41. "Oral Polio Vaccine," Global Polio Eradication Initiative, http://www .polioeradication.org/Polioandprevention/Thevaccines/Oralpolio vaccine(OPV).aspx.

42. "People and Discoveries—Jonas Salk," A Science Odyssey, PBS.org, 2010, http://www.pbs.org/wgbh/aso/databank/entries/bmsalk.html.

43. Sheryl Stolberg, "Jonas Salk, Whose Vaccine Conquered Polio, Dies at 80," Los Angeles Times, June 24, 1995, http://articles.latimes.com/1995-06 -24/news/mn-16682_1_first-polio-vaccine.

44. Richard D. Heffner, "Man Evolving . . . an Interview with Jonas Salk," Open Mind, May 11, 1985, http://www.thirteen.org/openmind-archive /science/man-evolving/.

Epilogue

1. Mark Joseph Stern, "Listen to Reagan's Press Secretary Laugh About Gay People Dying of AIDS," Slate, December 1, 2015, http://www.slate.com /blogs/outward/2015/12/01/reagan_press_secretary_laughs_about_gay _people_dying_of_aids.html.

2. Ronald Reagan, "The President's News Conference—September 17, 1985," https://reaganlibrary.archives.gov/archives/speeches/1985/91785c .htm.

3. Hank Plante, "Reagan's Legacy," HIV Info—Hot Topics—from the Experts, San Francisco AIDS Foundation, 2011, http://sfaf.org/hiv-info/hot-topics /from-the-experts/2011-02-reagans-legacy.html?referrer=https://www .google.com/.

4. William F. Buckley Jr., "Crucial Steps in Combating the Aids Epidemic; Identify All the Carriers," New York Times, op-ed, March 18, 1986, https://www.nytimes.com/books/00/07/16/specials/buckley-aids.html.

5. William Martin, With God on Our Side: The Rise of the Religious Right in America (New York: Broadway Books, 1996), p. 248.

6. "Huckabee Wanted AIDS Patients Isolated," *Los Angeles Times*, December 9, 2007, http://articles.latimes.com/2007/dec/09/nation/na -huckabee9.

7. "Mike Huckabee Advocated Isolation of AIDS Patients in 1992 Senate Race," Fox News, December 8, 2007, http://www.foxnews.com/story/2007 /12/08/mike-huckabee-advocated-isolation-aids-patients-in-12-senate -race.html.

8. Catherine Shoard, "Elizabeth Taylor 'Worth up to 1Bn' at Time of Death," *Guardian*, March 29, 2011, http://www.theguardian.com/film/2011/mar /29/elizabeth-taylor-worth-1bn-death.

9. David Aikman, *Billy Graham: His Life and Influence* (Nashville: Thomas Nelson, 2007), p. 261.

10. John Morrison, *Mathilde Krim and the Story of AIDS* (New York: Chel-sea House, 2004), Kindle edition, excerpt, p. 57, https://books.google .com/books?id=K-ZU35x2JaoC&pg=PA54&lpg=PA54&dq=How+much +did+government+spend+investigating+tylenol&source=bl&ots =MYVv0GgLiT&sig=aGgVsBpQN6ItG971z4EFlEjqaQ8&hl=en&sa=X &ved=0ahUKEwjBlLmwxrTMAhVDdj4KHQFKB00Q6AEILDAC#v =onepage&q=How%20much%20did%20government%20spend%20 investigating%20tylenol&f=false.

11. "Catholics, Condoms and AIDS," *New York Times*, October 20, 1989, http://www.nytimes.com/1989/10/20/opinion/catholics-condoms-and -aids.html.

12. David Koon, "Ruth Coker Burks, the Cemetery Angel," *Arkansas Times*, January 8, 2015.

13. Stefan Zweig, *The World of Yesterday* (1943; reprint, Lexington, MA: Plun-kett Lake Press, 2011), p. 5.

Sources

Antonine Plague

Birley, Anthony R. *Marcus Aurelius: A Biography*. New York: Routledge, 2000.

Boak, Arthur Edward Romilly. *A History of Rome to 565 AD*. New York: Macmillan, 1921. Kindle edition.

Cicero, Marcus Tullius. *The Orations of Marcus Tullius Cicero*. Translated by C. D. Young. 1851. University of Toronto, Robarts Library archives.

D'Aulaire, Edgar Parin, and Ingri D'Aulaire. *D'Aulaires' Book of Greek Myths*. New York: Delacorte Press, 1962.

Dio, Cassius. *Roman History*. Loeb Classical Library. Cambridge, MA: Harvard University Press, 1911.

Fears, J. Rufus. "The Plague Under Marcus Aurelius and the Decline and Fall of the Roman Empire." *Infectious Disease Clinics* 18, no. 1 (March 2004). http://www.id.theclinics.com/article/S0891-5520(03)00089-8/abstract.

Forbush, William Byron, ed. *Fox's Book of Martyrs: A History of the Lives, Sufferings and Triumphant Deaths of the Early Christian and Protestant Martyrs*. Philadelphia: John C. Winston, 1926.

"Germanic Peoples." *Encyclopedia Britannica*. http://www.britannica.com/topic/Germanic-peoples.

Gibbon, Edward. *The History of the Decline and Fall of the Roman Empire*. New York: Dutton, 1910.

Grant, Michael. *The Antonines: The Roman Empire in Transition*. London: Routledge, 1994.

Hinds, Kathryn. *Everyday Life in the Roman Empire*. New York: Cavendish Square, 2009.

Kohn, George Childs, ed. *Encyclopedia of Plague and Pestilence: From Ancient Times to the Present*. 3rd ed. New York: Facts on File, 2008.

Maire, Brigitte, ed. *"Greek" and "Roman" in Latin Medical Texts: Studies in Cultural Change and Exchange in Ancient Medicine*. Leiden: Brill, 2014.

Marcus Aurelius. *The Meditations of Marcus Aurelius Antoninus*. Edited by

A. S. L. Farquharson. Oxford: Oxford University Press (Oxford World's Classics), 2008.

"Marcus Aurelius Biography." Biography.com. http://www.biography.com/people/marcus-aurelius-9192657#challenges-to-his-authority.

Mattern, Susan P. *Galen and the Rhetoric of Healing.* Baltimore: Johns Hopkins University Press, 2008.

McLynn, Frank. *Marcus Aurelius: A Life.* Cambridge, MA: Da Capo Press, 2009.

Niebuhr, Barthold Georg. *Lectures on the History of Rome: From the First Punic War to the Death of Constantine.* 1844. E-source courtesy of Getty Research Institute. https://archive.org/details/historyofrome01nieb.

Phang, Sara Elise. *The Marriage of Roman Soldiers (13 B.C.–A.D. 235): Law and Family in the Imperial Army.* New York: Trustees of Columbia University, 2001.

Raoult, Didier, and Michel Drancourt, eds. *Paleomicrobiology: Past Human Infections.* Berlin: Springer-Verlag, 2008.

"Roman Freedmen." Quatr.us. 2016. http://www.historyforkids.org/learn/romans/people/freedmen.htm#.

Scheidel, Walter. "Marriage, Families, and Survival in the Roman Imperial Army: Demographic Aspects." Princeton/Stanford Working Papers in Classics, Stanford University, 2005. https://www.princeton.edu/~pswpc/pdfs/scheidel/110509.pdf.

Sheppard, John George. *The Fall of Rome and the Rise of the New Nationalities: A Series of Lectures on the Connections Between Ancient and Modern History.* New York: Routledge, 1892. University of Toronto, Robarts Library archives, https://archive.org/details/fallofromeriseof00shepuoft.

Tacitus. *Complete Works of Tacitus.* New York: McGraw-Hill, 1964.

Thatcher, Oliver J., ed. *The Library of Original Sources.* Vol. 4, *Early Mediaeval Age.* 1901. Reprint, Honolulu: University Press of the Pacific, 2004.

Thucydides. *History of the Peloponnesian War.* Translated by Richard Crawley. New York: Dutton, 1910.

Vesalius, Andreas. *On the Fabric of the Human Body.* Translated by W. F. Richardson and J. B. Carman. San Francisco: Norman, 1998–2009.

Bubonic Plague

Aberth, John. *From the Brink of the Apocalypse: Confronting Famine, War, Plague and Death in the Later Middle Ages.* London: Routledge, 2001.

Alden, Henry Mills, ed. "The Great Epidemics." *Harper's New Monthly Magazine,* June to November 1856. Internet Archive 2013. https://archive.org/details/harpersnew13harper.

Bailey, Diane. *The Plague (Epidemics and Society).* New York: Rosen, 2010.

Benedictow, Ole. J. "The Black Death: The Greatest Catastrophe Ever." *History Today* 55, no. 3 (March 2005). http://www.historytoday.com/ole-j-benedictow/black-death-greatest-catastrophe-ever.

"Black Death." History website. http://www.history.com/topics/black-death.

"The Black Death." BBC Bitesize Key Stage 3 website. http://www.bbc.co.uk /bitesize/ks3/history/middle_ages/the_black_death/revision/5/.

"The Black Death." In SlideShare, July 15, 2008. http://www.slideshare.net /guest13e41f/black-death-514058.

Boccaccio, Giovanni. *The Decameron*. Translated by John Payne. New York: Walter J. Black, 2007. Project Gutenberg e-Book. https://www.gutenberg .org/files/23700/23700-h/23700-h.htm.

Cantor, Norman F. *In The Wake of the Plague*. New York: HarperCollins, 2003.

Deary, Terry. *Horrible History: The Measly Middle Age*. Scholastic, 2015.

"The Flagellants' Attempt to Repel the Black Death, 1349." EyeWitness to History.com. 2010. http://www.eyewitnesstohistory.com/flagellants.htm.

Gottfried, Robert S. *The Black Death: Natural and Human Disaster in Medieval Europe*. New York: Free Press, 1983.

Haydn, Terry, and Christine Counsell, eds. *History, ICT and Learning in the Secondary School*. London: Routledge, 2003.

Kallen, Stuart A. *Prophecies and Soothsayers (The Mysterious & Unknown)*. San Diego: Reference Point Press, 2011.

Kelly, John. *The Great Mortality*. New York: HarperCollins, 2005. Kindle edition.

Leasor, James. *The Plague and the Fire*. Thirsk: House of Stratus, 2001.

Mitchell, Linda E., Katherine L. French, and Douglas L. Biggs, eds. "The Ties that Bind: Essays in Medieval British History in Honor of Barbara Hannawalt." *History: The Journal of the Historical Association*, 96, no. 324 (September 9, 2011). http://onlinelibrary.wiley.com/doi/10.1111/j.1468 -229X.2011.00531_2.x/abstract.

"Myths About Onion." National Onion Association website. http://www .onions-usa.org/faqs/onion-flu-cut-myths.

"Newcomers Facts." National Geographic Channel, October 25, 2013. http:// channel.nationalgeographic.com/meltdown/articles/newcomers-facts/.

"Nostradamus." *Encyclopedia of World Biography*. http://www.notablebio graphies.com/Ni-Pe/Nostradamus.html.

"Nostradamus Biography." Biography.com. http://www.biography.com/peo ple/nostradamus-9425407#studies.

"Nostradamus Was the Most Famous Plague Doctor During Black Death Years." Pravda Report, pravda.ru website, February 9, 2009. http://english .pravda.ru/science/earth/09-02-2009/107080-nostradamus_black _death-0/.

Pahl, Ronald Hans. *Creative Ways to Teach the Mysteries of History*. Vol. 1. Lanham, MD: Rowman and Littlefield Education, 2005.

"Petrarch on the Plague." The Decameron Web, a project of the Italian Studies Department's Virtual Humanities Lab at Brown University, February 18, 2010. http://www.brown.edu/Departments/Italian_Studies/dweb/pla gue/perspectives/petrarca.php.

"Plague—Fact Sheet No. 267." World Health Organization media website, November 2014. http://www.who.int/mediacentre/factsheets/fs267/en/.

"Rat-Shit-Covered Physicians Baffled by Spread of Black Plague." *Onion*, December 15, 2009. http://www.theonion.com/article/rat-shit-covered -physicians-baffled-by-spread-of-b-2876.

Roberts, Russell. *The Life and Times of Nostradamus*. Hockessin, DE: Mitchell Lane, 2008.

Ross, Scarlett. *Nostradamus for Dummies*. Hoboken, NJ: Wiley, 2005.

Slavicek, Louise Chipley. *Great Historic Disasters: The Black Death*. New York: Chelsea House, 2008.

Trendacosta, Katherine. "The 'Science' Behind Today's Plague Doctor Costume." iO9blog. October 19, 2015. http://io9.gizmodo.com/the-science -behind-todays-plague-doctor-costume-1737404375.

Wilson, Ian. *Nostradamus: The Man Behind the Prophecies*. New York: St. Martin's Press, 2002.

Dancing Plague

Backman, E. Louis. *Religious Dances*. Translated by E. Classen. Alton, UK: Dance Books, 2009.

Berger, Fred K. "Conversion Disorder." Medline Plus. October 31, 2014. https://www.nlm.nih.gov/medlineplus/ency/article/000954.htm.

"Cases of Mass Hysteria Throughout History." Onlineviralnews.com. September 18, 2015. http://onlineviralnews.com/cases-of-mass-hysteria-throughout -history/.

"Contagious Laughter." WYNC RadioLab. Season 4, episode 1. http://www .radiolab.org/story/91595-contagious-laughter/.

Dominus, Susan, "What Happened to the Girls in Le Roy." *New York Times Magazine*. March 7, 2012. http://www.nytimes.com/2012/03/11/magazine /teenage-girls-twitching-le-roy.html.

Kramer, Heinrich, and James (Jacob) Sprenger. *Malleus Maleficarum*. 1486. Translated by Montague Summers in 1928. Digireads.com. 2009.

Mendelson, Scott. "Conversion Disorder and Mass Hysteria." *Huffpost Healthy Living*, February 2, 2012. http://www.huffingtonpost.com/scott -mendelson-md/mass-hysteria_b_1239012.html.

Midelfort, H. C. Erik. *A History of Madness in Sixteenth-Century Germany*. Stanford: Stanford University Press, 1999.

Paracelsus. *Essential Theoretical Writings*. Edited by Wouter J. Hanegraaff. Translated by Andrew Weeks. Leiden: Brill, 2008. http://selfdefinition.org /magic/Paracelsus-Essential-Theoretical-Writings.pdf.

Sebastian, Simone. "Examining 1962's 'Laughter Epidemic.'" *Chicago Tribune*, July 29, 2003. http://articles.chicagotribune.com/2003-07-29/features/0307 290281_1_laughing-40th-anniversary-village.

Siegel, Lee. "Cambodians' Vision Loss Linked to War Trauma." *Los Angeles*

Times, October 15, 1989. http://articles.latimes.com/1989-10-15/news/mn
-232_1_vision-loss.

"St. Vitus' Dance." BBC Radio 3. September 7, 2012. http://www.bbc.co.uk
/programmes/b018h8kv.

Waller, John. *The Dancing Plague: The Strange, True Story of an Extraordinary Illness.* Naperville, IL: Sourcebooks, 2009.

———. "In a Spin: The Mysterious Dancing Epidemic of 1518." *Science Direct,* September 2008. http://www.sciencedirect.com/science/article/pii/S0160
932708000379.

Smallpox

Bell, John. *Bell's British Theatre, Consisting of the Most Esteemed English Plays.* Vol. 17. 1780. Google digital from the library of Harvard University. https://archive.org/details/bellsbritishthe19bellgoog.

Bingham, Jane. *The Inca Empire.* Chicago: Reed Elsevier, 2007.

Boseley, Sarah. "Lancet Retracts 'Utterly False' MMR Paper." *Guardian,* February 2, 2010. http://www.theguardian.com/society/2010/feb/02/lancet
-retracts-mmr-paper.

Buckley, Christopher. *But Enough About You.* New York: Simon and Schuster, 2014.

Campbell, John. "An Account of the Spanish Settlements in America." 1762. Hathi Trust Digital Library. http://catalog.hathitrust.org/Record/008
394522.

Clark, Liesl. "The Sacrificial Ceremony." *NOVA.* November 24, 1998. http://
www.pbs.org/wgbh/nova/ancient/sacrificial-ceremony.html.

"The Conquest of the Incas—Francisco Pizarro." PBS.org. http://www.pbs
.org/conquistadors/pizarro/pizarro_flat.html.

Cook, Noble David. *Born to Die: Disease and New World Conquest, 1492–1650.* Cambridge: Cambridge University Press, 1998.

Deer, Brian. "Exposed: Andrew Wakefield and the MMR-Autism Fraud." briandeer.com. http://briandeer.com/mmr/lancet-summary.htm.

———. "MMR Doctor Given Legal Aid Thousands." *Sunday Times,* December 31, 2006. http://briandeer.com/mmr/st-dec-2006.htm.

Diamond, Jared M. *Guns, Germs and Steel: The Fates of Human Societies.* New York: Norton, 1997.

———. "Episode One: Out of Eden—Transcript." *Guns, Germs and Steel.* ETV Education, PBS.org. 2016 http://www.pbs.org/gunsgermssteel/show
/transcript1.html.

"The Fall of the Aztecs—December 1520: Siege, Starvation & Smallpox." PBS
.org. http://www.pbs.org/conquistadors/cortes/cortes_h00.html.

"Frequently Asked Questions about Smallpox Vaccine." Centers of Disease Control and Prevention. http://www.bt.cdc.gov/agent/smallpox/vacci
nation/faq.asp.

Gordon, Richard. *The Alarming History of Medicine*. New York: St. Martin's Griffin, 1993.

Grob, Gerald N. *The Deadly Truth: A History of Disease in America*. Cambridge, MA: Harvard University Press, 2005.

Gross, C. P., and K. A. Sepkowitz. "The Myth of the Medical Breakthrough: Smallpox, Vaccination, and Jenner Reconsidered." *International Journal of Infectious Diseases*, July 1998. https://www.researchgate.net/publication/13454451_Gross_CP_Sepkowitz_KAThe_myth_of_the_medical_breakthrough_smallpox_vaccination_and_Jenner_reconsidered_Int_J_Infect_Dis_354-60.

Grundy, Isobel. *Lady Mary Wortley Montagu: Comet of the Enlightenment*. Oxford: Oxford University Press, 1999.

Halsall, Paul. "Modern History Sourcebook: Lady Mary Wortley Montagu (1689–1762): Smallpox Vaccination in Turkey." Fordham University, July 1998. http://legacy.fordham.edu/halsall/mod/montagu-smallpox.asp.

"Human Sacrifice and Cannibalism in the Aztec People." Michigan State University, Rise of Civilization course, April 21, 2013. http://anthropology.msu.edu/anp363-ss13/2013/04/21/human-sacrifice-and-cannibalism-in-the-aztec-people/.

Jakobsen, Hanne. "The Epidemic That Was Wiped Out." ScienceNordic, April 14, 2012. http://sciencenordic.com/epidemic-was-wiped-out.

Jongko, Paul. "10 Ancient Cultures That Practiced Ritual Human Sacrifice." TopTenz website: July 29, 2014. http://www.toptenz.net/10-ancient-cultures-practiced-ritual-human-sacrifice.php-.

Kramer, Samantha. "Aztec Human Sacrifice." Michigan State University, Great Discoveries in Archaeology course, April 25, 2013. http://anthropology.msu.edu/anp264-ss13/2013/04/25/aztec-human-sacrifice/.

MacQuarrie, Kim. *The Last Days of the Incas*. New York: Simon and Schuster, 2007.

Mann, Charles C. "1491." *Atlantic*, March 2002. http://www.theatlantic.com/magazine/archive/2002/03/1491/302445/.

"Measles." Media Center—Fact Sheet. World Health Organization. March 2016. http://www.who.int/mediacentre/factsheets/fs286/en/.

Montagu, Lady Mary Wortley. "Lady Mary Wortley Montagu on Small Pox in Turkey [Letter]." Annotated by Lynda Payne. Children and Youth in History. Item #157. https://chnm.gmu.edu/cyh/primary-sources/157.

Oldstone, Michael B. A. *Viruses, Plagues and History*. Oxford: Oxford University Press, 1998. The *New York Times* on the Web—Books. https://www.nytimes.com/books/first/o/oldstone-viruses.html.

Osler, William. "Man's Redemption of Man." *American Magazine*, November 2010 to April 1911. Digitized by Google. https://books.google.com/books?id=I-EvAAAAMAAJ&pg=PA251&lpg=PA251&dq=Here+I+would+like+to+say+a+word+or+two+upon+one+of+the+most+terrible+of+all+acute+infections,+the+one+of+which+we+first+learned+the+control+thr

ough+the+work+of+Jenner.+A+great+deal+of+literature+has+been+di
stributed&source=bl&ots=ijHGbb6zsT&sig=FbS0JbRnrwolCKqaOt-
dRLKxSYeg&hl=en&sa=X&ved=0ahUKEwjoqqHooavMAhWHtYMK
HU6yB3UQ6AEIHTAA#v=onepage&q=Here%20I%20would%20
like%20to%20say%20a%20word%20or%20two%20upon%20one%20
of%20the%20most%20terrible%20of%20all%20acute%20infec
tions%2C%20the%20one%20of%20which%20we%20first%20
learned%20the%20control%20through%20the%20work%20of%20Jen
ner.%20A%20great%20deal%20of%20literature%20has%20been%20dis
tributed&f=false.

Pringle, Heather. "Lofty Ambitions of the Inca." *National Geographic*, April 2011. http://ngm.nationalgeographic.com/2011/04/inca-empire/pringle-text/1.

Riedel, Stefan. "Edward Jenner and the History of Smallpox and Vaccination." Baylor University Medical Center Proceedings, January 2005. http://www.ncbi.nlm.nih.gov/pmc/articles/PMC1200696/.

Rotberg, Robert I., ed. *Health and Disease in Human History*. A Journal of Interdisciplinary History Reader. Cambridge, MA: MIT Press, 1953.

Salcamayhua, Don Juan. "An Account of the Antiquities of Peru." Sacred-Texts.com. http://www.sacred-texts.com/nam/inca/rly/rly2.htm.

Shuttleton, David E. *Smallpox and the Literary Imagination, 1660–1820*. Cambridge: Cambridge University Press, 2007.

Stevenson, Mark. "Brutality of Aztecs, Mayas Corroborated." *Los Angeles Times*, January 23, 2005. http://articles.latimes.com/2005/jan/23/news/adfg-sacrifice23.

"The Story of . . . Smallpox—and Other Deadly Eurasian Germs." From *Guns, Germs and Steel*. PBS.org. http://www.pbs.org/gunsgermssteel/variables/smallpox.html.

"Timeline of Germ Warfare." ABC News. http://abcnews.go.com/Nightline/story?id=128610.

"Variolation." Project Gutenberg Self-Publishing Press. http://self.gutenberg.org/articles/variolation.

Viegas, Jennifer. "Aztecs: Cannibalism Confirmed?" *Tribe*, January 28, 2005. http://history-geeks-get-chicks.tribe.net/thread/a46bf658-ce68-4840-93 a6-c10f66302485.

Whipps, Heather. "How Smallpox Changed the World." Livescience website. June 23, 2008. http://www.livescience.com/7509-smallpox-changed-world.html.

Wood, Michael. *Conquistadors*. BBC Digital. 2015. https://books.google.com/books?id=xKqFCAAAQBAJ&pg=PA90&lpg=PA90&dq=%22Cort%C3 %A9s+stared+at+him+for+a+moment+and+then+patted+him+on+the +head.%22&source=bl&ots=eTKqshNJKf&sig=gtnbajA3wRSChgmOF WsJgRTdGPc&hl=en&sa=X&ved=0CCYQ6AEwAWoVChMIivn7vODl xgIV1FmICh3E5QPM#v=onepage&q=smallpox&f=false.

Syphilis

Blackmon, Kayla Jo. "Public Power, Private Matters: The American Social Hygiene Association and the Policing of Sexual Health in the Progressive Era." Thesis, University of Montana, Missoula, MT. May 2014. http://etd .lib.umt.edu/theses/available/etd-06262014-081201/unrestricted/public powerprivatemattersblackmanthesisupload.pdf.

Blackwood's Edinburgh Magazine, April 1818. Ann Arbor: University of Michigan Library, 2009. https://books.google.com/books?id=res7AQA AMAAJ&pg=PA554&lpg=PA554&dq=No+Nose+club+edin burgh+magazine&source=bl&ots=W4wo-3O32h&sig=uIMQ aVaBbfUR2jhEGvRsl_GWZZ4&hl=en&sa=X&ved=0ahUKEwijzYSmx 57MAhVG3mMKHRQ9AkEQ6AEIMjAD#v=onepage&q=No%20 Nose%20club%20edinburgh%20magazine&f=false.

Chahal, Vickram. "The Evolution of Nasal Reconstruction: The Origins of Plastic Surgery." Proceedings of the 10th Annual History of Medicine Days. University of Calgary, Calgary, Alberta, March 23–24, 2001. http:// www.ucalgary.ca/uofc/Others/HOM/Dayspapers2001.pdf.

Conrad, Lawrence I., Michael Neve, Vivian Nutton, Roy Porter, and Andrew Wear. *The Western Medical Tradition: 800 BC to AD 1800.* Cambridge: Cambridge University Press, 1995.

"Diseases and Conditions: Syphilis." Mayo Clinic. January 2, 2014. http:// www.mayoclinic.org/diseases-conditions/syphilis/basics/symptoms /con-20021862.

Eamon, William. *The Professor of Secrets: Mystery, Medicine, and Alchemy in Renaissance Italy.* Washington: National Geographic Society, 2010.

Fitzharris, Lindsey. "Renaissance Rhinoplasty: The 16th-Century Nose Job." The Chirurgeon's Apprentice website. September 4, 2013. http://the chirurgeonsapprentice.com/2013/09/04/renaissance-rhinoplasty-the -16th-century-nose-job/#f1.

Frith, John. "Syphilis—Its Early History and Treatment until Penicillin and the Debate on Its Origins." *Journal of Military and Veterans' Health* 20, no. 4 (). http://jmvh.org/article/syphilis-its-early-history-and-treatment -until-penicillin-and-the-debate-on-its-origins/.

Hayden, Deborah. *Pox: Genius, Madness and the Mysteries of Syphilis.* New York: Basic Books, 2003.

Hertz, Abraham, and Emanuel Lincoln. *The Hidden Lincoln: From the Letters and Papers of William H. Herndon.* New York: Viking Press, 1938.

Jordan, Anne. *Love Well the Hour: The Life of Lady Colin Campbell, 1857–1911.* Leicester: Matador, 2010.

Jung, C. G. *Nietzsche's Zarathustra: Notes of the Seminar given in 1934–1939.* 2 vols. Edited by James L. Jarrett. Princeton: Princeton University Press, 2012. E-book.

Magner, Lois N. *A History of Medicine*. New York: Marcel Dekker, 1992.

Matthews, Robert. "'Madness' of Nietzsche Was Cancer Not Syphilis." *Telegraph*, May 4, 2003. http://www.telegraph.co.uk/education/3313279/Madness-of-Nietzsche-was-cancer-not-syphilis.html.

"Nasal Reconstruction Using a Paramedian Forehead Flap." Wikipedia. July 22, 2014. http://en.wikipedia.org/wiki/Nasal_reconstruction_using_a_paramedian_forehead_flap#cite_note-2.

Rotunda, A. M., and R. G. Bennett. "The Forehead Flap for Nasal Reconstruction: How We Do It." Skin Therapy Letter.com. March 2006. http://www.skintherapyletter.com/2006/11.2/2.html.

Serratore, Angela. "Lady Colin: The Victorian Not-Quite-Divorcee Who Scandalized London." Jezebel.com. November 11, 2014. http://jezebel.com/lady-colin-the-victorian-not-quite-divorcee-who-scanda-1650034397.

Sinclair, Upton. *Damaged Goods*: John C. Winston Company, 1913.

Stapelberg, Monica-Maria. *Through the Darkness: Glimpses into the History of Western Medicine*. UK: Crux, 2016.

Stewart, Walter. *Nietzsche: My Sister and I: A Critical Study*. Xlibris, 2007.

Weiss, Philip. "Beethoven's Hair Tells All!" *New York Times Magazine*, November 29, 1998. http://www.nytimes.com/1998/11/29/magazine/beethoven-s-hair-tells-all.html?pagewanted=all.

Tuberculosis

Brown, Sue. *Joseph Severn, A Life: The Rewards of Friendship*. Oxford: Oxford University Press, 2009.

Bynum, Helen. *Spitting Blood: The History of Tuberculosis*. Oxford: Oxford University Press, 2012.

Byrne, Katherine. *Tuberculosis and the Victorian Literary Imagination*. Cambridge: Cambridge University Press, 2011.

Clark, James. *Medical Notes on Climate, Diseases, Hospitals, and Medical Schools, in France, Italy and Switzerland*. 1820, Reprint, Cambridge: Cambridge University Press, 2013.

Dubos, Rene, and Jean Dubos. *The White Plague: Tuberculosis, Man and Society*. Boston: Little, Brown, 1996.

Frith, John. "History of Tuberculosis: Part 1—Phthisis, Consumption and the White Plague." *Journal of Military and Veterans' Health* 22, no. 2 (November 2012). http://jmvh.org/article/history-of-tuberculosis-part-1-phthisis-consumption-and-the-white-plague/.

Hawksley, Lucinda. *Lizzie Siddal: The Tragedy of a Pre-Raphaelite Supermodel*. New York: Walker, 2004.

Hugo, Victor. *The Works of Victor Hugo, One Volume Edition*. New York: Collier, 1928.

"International Drug Price Indicator Guide—Vaccine, Bcg." Management Sciences for Health. 2014. http://erc.msh.org/dmpguide/resultsdetail.cfm?language=english&code=BCG00A&s_year=2014&year=2014&str

=&desc=Vaccine%2C%20BCG&pack=new&frm=POWDER&rte=INJ &class_code2=19%2E3%2E&supplement=&class_name=%2819%2E3% 2E%29Vaccines%3Cbr%3E.

Jeaffreson, John Cordy. *The Real Lord Byron: New Views of the Poet's Life*. Vol. 2. Ann Arbor: University of Michigan Library, 1883 (reprint 2012).

Keats, John. *The Letters of John Keats: Volume 2*. Edited by Hyder Edward Rollins. Cambridge, MA: Harvard University Press, 1958.

Lawlor, Clark. *Consumption and Literature: The Making of the Romantic Disease*. New York: Palgrave Macmillan, 2007.

Marshall, Henrietta Elizabeth. *Uncle Tom's Cabin Told to the Children*. From the Told to the Children series, edited by Louey Chisholm. New York: Dutton, 1904. http://utc.iath.virginia.edu/childrn/cbjackhp .html.

McLean, Hugh. *In Quest of Tolstoy*. Boston: Academic Studies Press, 2010.

Poe, Edgar Allan. *Great Short Works of Edgar Allan Poe*. Edited by G. R. Thompson. New York: Harper Collins, 1970.

Risse, Guenter B. *New Medical Challenges During the Scottish Enlightenment*. Leiden: Brill, 2005.

Roe, Nicholas. *John Keats: A New Life*. New Haven, CT: Yale University Press, 2012.

"Tuberculosis." Centers for Disease Control and Prevention. December 9, 2011. http://www.cdc.gov/tb/topic/treatment/.

"What Is Tuberculosis?" National Institute of Allergy and Infectious Diseases. March 6, 2009. http://www.niaid.nih.gov/topics/tuberculosis /understanding/whatistb/Pages/default.aspx.

Whitney, Daniel H. *The Family Physician, and Guide to Health, Together with the History, Causes, Symptoms and Treatment of the Asiatic Cholera, a Glossary Explaining the Most Difficult Words That Occur in Medical Science, and a Copious Index, to Which Is Added an Appendix*. 1833. U.S. National Library of Medicine website. https://archive.org/details /2577008R.nlm.nih.gov.

Cholera

Dickens, Charles. "The Troubled Water Question." *Household Words, a Weekly Journal*, April 13, 1850. https://books.google.com/books?id=MPNAAQAA MAAJ&pg=PA53&lpg=PA53&dq=charles+dickens+troubled+water+ques tion&source=bl&ots=aVNLBwQOCh&sig=oAGlhCUH9fzUJik8ll HyOxoCjSI&hl=en&sa=X&ved=0ahUKEwiho5uK8OHLAhWBbiYKHV 5iChkQ6AEILTAD#v=onepage&q=charles%20dickens%20troubled%20 water%20question&f=false.

Dorling, Danny. *Unequal Health: The Scandal of Our Times*. Bristol: Policy Press, 2013.

Halliday, Stephen. "Death and Miasma in Victorian London: An Obstinate

Belief." *British Medical Journal*, October 23, 2001. http://www.bmj.com/content/323/7327/1469.

———. *The Great Stink of London: Sir Joseph Bazalgette and the Cleansing of the Victorian Metropolis*. Gloucestershire: History Press, 2001.

Hempel, Sandra. "John Snow." *Lancet* 381, no. 9874 (April 13, 2013). http://www.thelancet.com/journals/lancet/article/PIIS0140-6736(13)60830-2/fulltext?elsca1=TW.

Johnson, Steven. *The Ghost Map: The Story of London's Most Terrifying Epidemic—and How It Changed Science, Cities, and the Modern World.* New York: Penguin, 2006. Kindle edition.

———. "How the 'Ghost Map' Helped End a Killer Disease." TEDsalon. November 2006. https://www.ted.com/talks/steven_johnson_tours_the_ghost_map?language=en#t-59501.

"Retrospect of Cholera in the East of London." *Lancet*, 2 (September 29, 1866). https://books.google.com/books?id=SxxAAAAAcAAJ&pg=PA1317&lpg=PA1317&dq=The+Lancet+london+Cholera+in+the+east+of+london++September+29+1866&source=bl&ots=Z-bAnpDI5s&sig=ZgLRBf3W-znA2gzwsbgZAzmuQBlE&hl=en&sa=X&ved=0ahUKEwimtf-Ik-LLAhUDKCYKHQQ5DwUQ6AEIHDAA#v=onepage&q=The%20Lancet%20london%20Cholera%20in%20the%20east%20of%20london%20%20September%2029%201866&f=false.

Reuters. "Why Bad Smells Make You Gag." ABC Science. March 5, 2008. http://www.abc.net.au/science/articles/2008/03/05/2180489.htm.

"Reverend Henry Whitehead." UCLA Department of Epidemiology, School of Public Health. http://www.ph.ucla.edu/epi/snow/whitehead.html.

Snow, John. "John Snow's Teetotal Address." Spring 1836. From the British Temperance Advocate, 1888. UCLA Department of Epidemiology, School of Public Health. http://www.ph.ucla.edu/epi/snow/teetotal.html.

———. "Letter to the Right Honourable Sir Benjamin Hall, Bart., President of the General Board of Health." July 12, 1855. Original pamphlet courtesy of the Historical Library, Yale University Medical School. The John Snow Archive and Research Companion. http://johnsnow.matrix.msu.edu/work.php?id=15-78-5A.

———. "On Chloroform and Other Anaesthetics: Their Action and Administration." January 1, 1858. The Wood Library Museum. http://www.woodlibrarymuseum.org/ebooks/item/643/snow,-john.-on-chloroform-and-other-anaesthetics,-their-action-and-administration-(with-a-memoir-of-the-author,-by-benjamin-w.-richardson).

———. "On the Mode of Communication of Cholera." Pamphlet. 1849. Reviewed in the *London Medical Gazette* 44 (September 14, 1849). The John Snow Archive and Research Companion. http://johnsnow.matrix.msu.edu/work.php?id=15-78-28.

"Snow's Testimony." UCLA Department of Epidemiology, School of Public Health. http://www.ph.ucla.edu/epi/snow/snows_testimony.html.

Tuthill, Kathleen. "John Snow and the Broad Street Pump." *Cricket*, November 2003. UCLA Department of Epidemiology, School of Public Health. http://www.ph.ucla.edu/epi/snow/snowcricketarticle.html.

Vinten-Johansen, Peter, Howard Brody, Nigel Paneth, Stephen Rachman, and Michael Rip. *Cholera, Chloroform, and the Science of Medicine: A Life of John Snow*. Oxford: Oxford University Press, 2003.

Leprosy

"An Act to Prevent the Spread of Leprosy, 1865." January 1865. National Park Service. http://www.nps.gov/kala/learn/historyculture/1865.htm.

"Appendix M: Special Report from Rev. J. Damien, Catholic Priest at Kalawao, March 1886." Report of the Board of Health. https://books.google.com /books?id=C7JNAAAAMAAJ&pg=PR110&lpg=PR110&dq=Spe cial+report+J.+Damien+1886&source=bl&ots=R1-cZ_SXPp&sig=M1D wLciA7V1IR-D-fKmCsPaen7I&hl=en&sa=X&ved=0ahUKEwj0-fvLsuLL AhWBLyYKHdSjArUQ6AEIKDAE#v=onepage&q=Special%20 report%20J.%20Damien%201886&f=false.

Blom, K. "Armauer Hansen and Human Leprosy Transmission. Medical Ethics and Legal Rights." 1973. U.S. National Library of Medicine. http://www .ncbi.nlm.nih.gov/pubmed/4592244.

Brown, Stephen. "Pope Canonizes Leper Saint Damien, Hailed by Obama." Edited by David Stamp. Reuters, October 11, 2009. http://www.reuters .com/article/2009/10/11/us-pope-saints-idUSTRE59A0YW20091011.

"Damien the Leper." Franciscans of St. Anthony's Guild. 1974. Eternal World Television Network. https://www.ewtn.com/library/MARY/DAMIEN .HTM.

Daws, Gavan. *Holy Man: Father Damien of Molokai*. Honolulu: University of Hawaii Press, 1989.

Eynikel, Hilde. *Molokai: The Story of Father Damien*. St. Paul's/Alba House, 1999.

Farrow, John. *Damien the Leper: A Life of Magnificent Courage, Devotion & Spirit*. New York: Image Books (Doubleday), 1954.

Gould, Tony. *A Disease Apart: Leprosy in the Modern World*. New York: St. Martin's Press, 2005.

O'Malley, Vincent J. *Saints of North America*. Huntington, IN: Our Sunday Visitor, 2004.

"St. Damien of Molokai." Catholic Online. http://www.catholic.org/saints /saint.php?saint_id=2817.

"Salmonella." Foodborne Illness website. http://www.foodborneillness.com /salmonella_food_poisoning/.

Senn, Nicholas. "Father Damien, the Leper Hero." *Journal of the American Medical Association*, August 27, 1904. https://books.google.com/books

?pg=PA605&lpg=PA607&sig=mJi_mLzilMWH9Ac7pkeCYkwZxXg&ei
=c6KySpScI9GklAe3y4H5Dg&ct=result&id=e-sBAAAAYAAJ&ots
=LaTpBrjyQJ#v=onepage&q&f=false.

Stevenson, Robert Louis. "Father Damien—an Open Letter to the Reverend
Dr. Hyde of Honolulu," February 25, 1890. http://www.fullbooks.com
/Father-Damien.html.

———. "The Letters of Robert Louis Stevenson—Volume 2, Letter to James Payn,
June 13, 1889." Free Books. http://robert-louis-stevenson.classic-literature
.co.uk/the-letters-of-robert-louis-stevenson-volume-2/ebook-page-60.as.

Stewart, Richard. *Leper Priest of Molokai: The Father Damien Story.* Honolulu:
University of Hawaii Press, 2000.

Volder, Jan de. *The Spirit of Father Damien: The Leper Priest—a Saint for Our
Time.* San Francisco: Ignatius Press, 2010.

Yandell, Kate. "The Leprosy Bacillus, circa 1873." *TheScientist,* October 1,
2013. http://www.the-scientist.com/?articles.view/articleNo/37619/title
/The-Leprosy-Bacillus—circa-1873/.

Typhoid

Baker, S. Josephine. *Fighting for Life.* 1939. Reprint, New York: New York
Times Review of Books, 2013.

Bartoletti, Susan Campbell. *Terrible Typhoid Mary: A True Story of the Deadliest Cook in America.* New York: Houghton Mifflin Harcourt, 2015.

Gray, Dr. Annie. "How to Make Ice Cream the Victorian Way." English Heritage website. http://www.english-heritage.org.uk/visit/pick-of-season
/how-to-make-victorian-ice-cream/.

Huber, John B. "'Microbe Carriers'—the Newly Discovered." *Richmond
Times-Dispatch,* July 11, 1915. Chronicling America: Historic American
Newspapers. Library of Congress. http://chroniclingamerica.loc.gov/lccn
/sn83045389/1915-07-11/ed-1/seq-42/#date1=1915&index=0&rows=20
&words=typhoid+Typhoid&searchType=basic&sequence=0&state=
&date2=1915&proxtext=typhoid&y=0&x=0&dateFilterType=year
Range&page=1.

Leavitt, Judith Walzer. *Typhoid Mary: Captive to the Public's Health.* Boston:
Beacon Press, 1996.

Lowth, Mary. "Typhoid and Paratyphoid Fever." Patient website. February 25,
2015. http://patient.info/doctor/typhoid-and-paratyphoid-fever-pro.

Mallon, Mary. "In Her Own Words." 2014, NOVA. http://www.pbs.org/wgbh
/nova/typhoid/letter.html.

McNeil, Donald G., Jr. "Bacteria Study Offers Clues to Typhoid Mary Mystery."
New York Times, August 26, 2013. http://www.nytimes.com/2013/08/27
/health/bacteria-study-offers-clues-to-typhoid-mary-mystery.html?_r=0.

"Mystery of the Poison Guest at Wealthy Mrs. Case's Party." *Richmond Times-
Dispatch,* August 22, 1920. Chronicling America: Historic American
Newspapers. Library of Congress. http://chroniclingamerica.loc.gov/lccn

/sn83045389/1920-08-22/ed-1/seq-51/#date1=1907&index=3&rows=20 &words=Mary+Typhoid+typhoid&searchType=basic&sequence =0&state=&date2=1922&proxtext=typhoid+mary+&y=12&x=1 &dateFilterType=yearRange&page=1.

Park, William H. "Typhoid Bacilli Carriers." 1908. Primary Sources: Workshops in American History. https://www.learner.org/workshops/primary sources/disease/docs/park2.html.

Petrash, Antonia. *More Than Petticoats: Remarkable New York Women.* Guilford, CT: TwoDot, 2001.

Sawyer, Wilbur A. "How a Dish of Baked Spaghetti Gave 93 Eaters Typhoid Fever." *Richmond Times Dispatch*, July 11, 1915. Chronicling America: Historic American Newspapers. Library of Congress. http://chroniclingamerica .loc.gov/lccn/sn83045389/1915-07-11/ed-1/seq-43/.

Soper, George A. "The Work of a Chronic Typhoid Germ Distributor." 1907. Primary Sources: Workshops in American History. https://www.learner .org/workshops/primarysources/disease/docs/soper2.html.

"Thrives on Typhoid." *Washington Herald*, April 7, 1907. Chronicling America: Historic American Newspapers. Library of Congress. http:// chroniclingamerica.loc.gov/lccn/sn83045433/1907-04-07/ed-1/seq-12/.

"Typhoid Mary Wants Liberty." *Richmond Planet*, July 10, 1909. Chronicling America: Historic American Newspapers. Library of Congress. http:// chroniclingamerica.loc.gov/lccn/sn84025841/1909-07-10/ed-1/seq-7 /#date1=1836&sort=relevance&rows=20&words=MARY+TYPHOID &searchType=basic&sequence=0&index=0&state=&date2=1922&prox text=typhoid+mary&y=0&x=0&dateFilterType=yearRange&page=2.

Spanish Flu

Barnett, Randy. "The Volokh Conspiracy: Expunging Woodrow Wilson from Official Places of Honor." *Washington Post*, June 25, 2015. https://www .washingtonpost.com/news/volokh-conspiracy/wp/2015/06/25 /expunging-woodrow-wilson-from-official-places-of-honor/.

Barry, John M. *The Great Influenza: The Story of the Deadliest Pandemic in History.* New York: Penguin, 2004.

Board of Global Health, Institute of Medicine of the National Academies. "The Threat of Pandemic Influenza: Are We Ready?" Workshop overview. National Center for Biotechnology Information. 2005. http://www.ncbi .nlm.nih.gov/books/NBK22148/.

——. *The Threat of Pandemic Influenza: Are We Ready?.* Workshop summary edited by Stacey L. Knobler, Alison Mack, Adel Mahmoud, Stanley M. Lemon. Washington: National Academies Press, 2005. http://www .ncbi.nlm.nih.gov/books/NBK22156/.

Connor, Steve. "American Scientists Controversially Recreate Deadly Spanish Flu." *Independent*, June 11, 2014. http://www.independent.co.uk

/news/science/american-scientists-controversially-recreate-deadly
-spanish-flu-virus-9529707.html.

Crosby, Alfred W. *America's Forgotten Pandemic: The Influenza of 1918*. Cambridge: Cambridge University Press, 2003. Kindle edition.

Dotinga, Randy. "5 Surprising Facts about Woodrow Wilson and Racism." *Christian Science Monitor*, December 14, 2013. http://www.csmonitor
.com/Books/chapter-and-verse/2015/1214/5-surprising-facts-about
-Woodrow-Wilson-and-racism.

Ewing, Tom. "Influenza in the News: Using Newspapers to Understand a Public Health Crisis." National Digital Newspaper—Program Awardee Conference, September 26, 2012. http://www.flu1918.lib.vt.edu/wp
-content/uploads/2012/11/NDNP_Ewing_Influenza_25Sept2012.pdf.

"The Flu of 1918." *Pennsylvania Gazette*, October 28, 1998. http://www.upenn
.edu/gazette/1198/lynch2.html.

"The Great Pandemic—New York." United States Department of Health and Human Services. http://www.flu.gov/pandemic/history/1918/your_state
/northeast/newyork/.

Greene, Jeffrey, and Karen Moline. *The Bird Flu Pandemic: Can It Happen? Will It Happen? How to Protect Your Family If It Does*. New York: St. Martin's Press, 2006.

Greenslade, Roy. "First World War: How State and Press Kept Truth off the Front Page." *Guardian*, July 27, 2014. http://www.theguardian.com/media
/2014/jul/27/first-world-war-state-press-reporting.

Hardy, Charles. " 'Please Let Me Put Him in a Macaroni Box'—the Spanish Influenza of 1918 in Philadelphia." WHYY-FM radio program *The Influenza Pandemic of 1918*. Philadelphia, 1984. History Matters website. http://historymatters.gmu.edu/d/13/.

"Influenza 1918." A complete transcript of the program. *American Experience*. PBS.org. 1998. http://www.pbs.org/wgbh/americanexperience/features
/transcript/influenza-transcript/.

Kolata, Gina. *The Story of the Great Influenza Pandemic of 1918 and the Search for the Virus That Caused It*. New York: Touchstone, 1999.

Kreiser, Christine M. "1918 Spanish Influenza Outbreak: The Enemy Within." HistoryNet website. October 27, 2006. http://www.historynet.com/1918
-spanish-influenza-outbreak-the-enemy-within.htm.

Nicholson, Juliet. "The War Was Over but Spanish Flu Would Kill Millions More." *Telegraph*, November 11, 2009. http://www.telegraph.co.uk/news
/health/6542203/The-war-was-over-but-Spanish-Flu-would-kill-mil
lions-more.html#disqus_thread.

"Over There." A song by George M. Cohan. Wikipedia. https://en.wikipedia
.org/wiki/Over_There.

Porter, Katharine Anne. *Pale Horse, Pale Rider: Three Short Novels*. New York: Harcourt Brace, 1967.

"Scientific Nursing Halting Epidemic." *Philadelphia Inquirer,* October 15, 1918. From the Influenza Encyclopedia, University of Michigan Library. http://quod.lib.umich.edu/f/flu/3990flu.0007.993/1.

"Spanish Influenza in North America, 1918–1919." Harvard University Library: Contagion—Historical Views of Diseases and Epidemics. http://ocp.hul.harvard.edu/contagion/influenza.html.

Trilla, Antoni, Guillem Trilla, and Carolyn Daer. "The 1918 'Spanish Flu' in Spain." *Oxford Journals, Clinical Infectious Diseases* 47, no. 5 (2008). http://cid.oxfordjournals.org/content/47/5/668.full.

Willerson, James T. "The Great Enemy—Infectious Disease." Edited by S. Ward Casscells and Mohammad Madjid. *Texas Heart Institute Journal,* 2004. http://www.ncbi.nlm.nih.gov/pmc/articles/PMC387424/.

"Woodrow Wilson." The Great Pandemic—The United States in 1918–1919. United States Department of Health and Human Services. http://www.flu.gov/pandemic/history/1918/biographies/wilson/.

Encephalitis Lethargica

Carswell, Sue. "Oliver Sacks." *People,* February 11, 1991. http://www.people.com/people/archive/article/0,20114432,00.html.

Crosby, Molly Caldwell. *Asleep: The Forgotten Epidemic That Remains One of Medicine's Greatest Mysteries.* New York: Berkley Books, 2010. Kindle edition.

Golden, Tim. "Bronx Doctor Has Best-Seller, Hit Movie and No Job." *New York Times,* February 16, 1991. http://www.nytimes.com/1991/02/16/nyregion/bronx-doctor-has-best-seller-hit-movie-and-no-job.html?pagewanted=all.

Kolata, Gina. *The Story of the Great Influenza Pandemic of 1918 and the Search for the Virus That Caused It.* New York: Touchstone, 1999.

"Mystery of the Forgotten Plague." BBC News. July 27, 2004. http://news.bbc.co.uk/2/hi/health/3930727.stm.

"Parkinson Disease." *New York Times Health Guide.* September 16, 2013. http://www.nytimes.com/health/guides/disease/parkinsons-disease/levadopa-(l-dopa).html.

Reid, Ann H., Sherman McCall, James M. Henry, and Jeffrey K. Taubenberger. "Experimenting on the Past: The Enigma of von Economo's Encephalitis Lethargica." *Journal of Neuropathology and Experimental Neurology,* July 2001. http://jnen.oxfordjournals.org/content/60/7/663.

Sacks, Oliver. *Awakenings.* New York: Vintage Books, 1999.

Vilensky, Joel A. *Encephalitis Lethargica: During and After the Epidemic.* Oxford: Oxford University Press, 2011. Kindle edition.

Vilensky, Joel A. "Sleeping Princes and Princesses: The Encephalitis Lethargica Epidemic of the 1920s and a Contemporary Evaluation of the Disease." Presentation Slides. 2008. http://slideplayer.com/slide/3899891/.

Vilensky, Joel A. "The 'Spanish Flu' Epidemic of 1918 & Encephalitis Lethargica." The Sophie Cameron Trust, Bath, England. http://www.thesophie camerontrust.org.uk/research-epedemic.htm.

Vincent, Angela. "Encephalitis Lethargica: Part of a Spectrum of Post-streptococcal Autoimmune Diseases?" *Brain: A Journal of Neurology*, December 16, 2003. http://brain.oxfordjournals.org/content/127/1/2.

Lobotomies

Beam, Alex. *Gracefully Insane: The Rise and Fall of America's Premier Mental Hospital*. New York: Public Affairs, 2009.

Borden, Audrey. *The History of Gay People in Alcoholics Anonymous: From the Beginning*. New York: Routledge, 2013.

Dully, Howard, and Charles Fleming. *My Lobotomy*. New York: Three Rivers Press, 2008.

Dynes, John B., and James L. Poppen. "Lobotomy for Intractable Pain." *Journal of the American Medical Association* 140, no. 1 (May 7, 1949). http://jama .jamanetwork.com/article.aspx?articleid=304291.

El-Hai, Jack. *The Lobotomist: A Maverick Medical Genius and His Tragic Quest to Rid the World of Mental Illness*. Hoboken, NJ: Wiley, 2005. Kindle edition.

Harkavy, Ward. "The Scary Days When Thousands Were Lobotomized on Long Island." *Village Voice*, October 26, 1999. http://www.villagevoice .com/long-island-voice/the-scary-days-when-thousands-were -lobotomized-on-long-island-7155435.

Harlow, John M. "Recovery from the Passage of an Iron Bar through the Head." Publications of the Massachusetts Medical Society, 1868. Wikisource. https://en.wikisource.org/wiki/Recovery_from_the_passage_of_an_iron _bar_through_the_head.

"Introduction: The Lobotomist." *American Experience*. PBS. http://www.pbs. org/wgbh/americanexperience/features/introduction/lobotomist -introduction/.

Kessler, Ronald. *The Sins of the Father: Joseph P. Kennedy and the Dynasty He Founded*. New York: Grand Central, 1996.

Kochar, Piya, and Dave Isay. "My Lobotomy: Howard Dully's Story." Edited by Gary Corvino. Sound Portraits Productions. NPR.org. November 16, 2005. http://www.npr.org/2005/11/16/5014080/my-lobotomy-howard-dullys -journey.

Larson, Kate Clifford. *Rosemary: The Hidden Kennedy Daughter*. New York: Houghton Mifflin Harcourt, 2015.

Levinson, Hugh. "The Strange and Curious History of Lobotomy." Magazine, BBC News, November 8, 2011. http://www.bbc.com/news/magazine -15629160.

"Lobotomy." PsychologistWorld.com. http://www.psychologistworld.com /biological/lobotomy.php.

Long, Tony. "Nov. 12, 1935: You Should (Not) Have a Lobotomy." WIRED, November 12, 2010. http://www.wired.com/2010/11/1112first-lobotomy/.

McGrath, Charles. "A Lobotomy That He Says Didn't Touch His Soul." *New York Times*, November 16, 2005. http://www.nytimes.com/2005/11/16 /arts/a-lobotomy-that-he-says-didnt-touch-his-soul.html.

"Moniz Develops Lobotomy for Mental Illness, 1935." People and Discoveries. ETV Education, PBS.org. http://www.pbs.org/wgbh/aso/databank /entries/dh35lo.html.

"My Lobotomy." *All Things Considered.* SoundPortraits Productions, November 16, 2005. http://soundportraits.org/on-air/my_lobotomy/transcript.php.

Phillips, Michael M. "The Lobotomy File, Part Two: One Doctor's Legacy." A *Wall Street Journal* special project. 2013. http://projects.wsj.com/lobo tomyfiles/?ch=two.

Pressman, Jack D. *Last Resort: Psychosurgery and the Limits of Medicine.* Edited by Charles Rosenberg and Colin James. Cambridge History of Medicine series. Cambridge: Cambridge University Press, 2002.

Raz, Mical. *Lobotomy Letters: The Making of American Psychosurgery.* Edited by Theodore M. Brown. Rochester Studies in Medical History series. Rochester, NY: University of Rochester Press, 2015.

Scull, Andrew T., ed. *Cultural Sociology of Mental Illness: An A-to-Z Guide.* Thousand Oaks, CA: Sage, 2014.

Vertosick, Frank T., Jr. "Lobotomy's Back." *Discover*, October 1997. http:// discovermagazine.com/1997/oct/lobotomysback1240.

Weiner, Eric. "Nobel Panel Urged to Rescind Prize for Lobotomies." NPR.org. August 10, 2005. http://www.npr.org/templates/story/story.php?storyId =4794007.

Polio

Castillo, Merrysha. "Jonas Salk." The Exercise of Leadership. Wagner College, New York. http://faculty.wagner.edu/lori-weintrob/jonas-salk/.

"Deadly Diseases: Polio." ETV Education, PBS.org. http://www.pbs.org/wgbh /rxforsurvival/series/diseases/polio.html.

"Double Party Held at Warm Springs." *New York Times*, January 30, 1934. http://query.nytimes.com/gst/abstract.html?res=9B01EED91E3DE23AB C4950DFB766838F629EDE.

Eisenhower, Dwight D. "Citation Presented to Dr. Jonas E. Salk and Accompanying Remarks." The American Presidency Project. April 22, 1955. http://www.presidency.ucsb.edu/ws/?pid=10457.

Heffner, Richard D. "Man Evolving . . . an Interview with Jonas Salk." *Open Mind*, May 11, 1985. http://www.thirteen.org/openmind-archive/science /man-evolving/.

Llanas, Sheila. *Jonas Salk: Medical Innovator and Polio Vaccine Developer.* Edina, MN: ABDO, 2013.

Loving, Sarah. "Herd Immunity (Community Immunity)." University of

Oxford, Vaccine Knowledge Project. http://www.ovg.ox.ac.uk/herd -immunity.

"Measles (MCV)—Data by Country." Global Health Observatory data repository. World Health Organization. http://apps.who.int/gho/data/node .main.A826?_ga=1.149767604.366030890.1401971125.

"Medicine: Closing In on Polio." *Time*, March 29, 1954. http://content.time .com/time/subscriber/article/0,33009,819686-4,00.html.

Musgrave, Ian. "'Toxins' in Vaccines: A Potentially Deadly Misunderstanding." *The Conversation*, November 28, 2012. http://theconversation.com /toxins-in-vaccines-a-potentially-deadly-misunderstanding-11010.

Nielsen, N. M., K. Rostgaard, K. Juel, D. Askgaard, and P. Aaby. "Long-term Mortality after Poliomyelitis." U.S. National Library of Medicine. May 2003. PubMed.com. http://www.ncbi.nlm.nih.gov/pubmed/12859038.

Offit, Paul A. *The Cutter Incident: How America's First Polio Vaccine Led to the Growing Vaccine Crisis*. New Haven, CT: Yale University Press, 2005. Kindle edition.

"Oral Polio Vaccine." Global Polio Eradication Initiative. http://www .polioeradication.org/Polioandprevention/Thevaccines/Oralpoliovaccine (OPV).aspx.

Oshinsky, David M. *Polio: An American Story*. Oxford: Oxford University Press, 2005.

"People and Discoveries—Jonas Salk." A Science Odyssey. PBS. org. http:// www.pbs.org/wgbh/aso/databank/entries/bmsalk.html.

Plotkin, Stanley. "'Herd Immunity': A Rough Guide." *Oxford Journals: Clinical Infectious Diseases* 52, no. 7 (2011). http://cid.oxfordjournals .org/content/52/7/911.full.

"Polio and Prevention." The Global Polio Eradication Initiative. http://www .polioeradication.org/polioandprevention.aspx.

"Polio: What You Need to Know." myDr website. January 12, 2011. http:// www.mydr.com.au/kids-teens-health/polio-what-you-need-to-know.

"Poliomyelitis." Fact Sheet No. 114. World Health Organization. October 2015. http://www.who.int/mediacentre/factsheets/fs114/en/.

Prabhu, Amar. "How Much Money Did Jonas Salk Potentially Forfeit by Not Patenting the Polio Vaccine?" *Forbes*, August 9, 2012. http://www.forbes .com/sites/quora/2012/08/09/how-much-money-did-jonas-salk -potentially-forfeit-by-not-patenting-the-polio-vaccine/#1e35e3941c2d.

Stolberg, Sheryl. "Jonas Salk, Whose Vaccine Conquered Polio, Dies at 80." *Los Angeles Times*, June 24, 1995. http://articles.latimes.com/1995-06-24 /news/mn-16682_1_first-polio-vaccine.

Thompson, Dennis. "The Salk Polio Vaccine: Greatest Public Health Experiment in History." CBS News, December 2, 2014. http://www.cbsnews.com/news /the-salk-polio-vaccine-greatest-public-health-experiment-in-history/.

Wilson, Daniel J. *Living with Polio: The Epidemic and Its Survivors*. Chicago: University of Chicago Press, 2005.

Epilogue

Aikman, David. *Billy Graham: His Life and Influence.* Nashville: Thomas Nelson, 2007.

Buckley, William F., Jr. "Crucial Steps in Combating the Aids Epidemic; Identify All the Carriers." *New York Times*, op-ed, March 18, 1986. https://www.nytimes.com/books/00/07/16/specials/buckley-aids.html.

"Catholics, Condoms and AIDS." *New York Times*, October 20, 1989. http://www.nytimes.com/1989/10/20/opinion/catholics-condoms-and-aids.html.

"Huckabee Wanted AIDS Patients Isolated." *Los Angeles Times*, December 9, 2007. http://articles.latimes.com/2007/dec/09/nation/na-huckabee9.

Martin, William. *With God on Our Side: The Rise of the Religious Right in America.* New York: Broadway Books, 1996.

"Mike Huckabee Advocated Isolation of AIDS Patients in 1992 Senate Race." Fox News. December 8, 2007. http://www.foxnews.com/story/2007/12/08/mike-huckabee-advocated-isolation-aids-patients-in-12-senate-race.html.

Morrison, John. *Mathilde Krim and the Story of AIDS.* New York: Chelsea House, 2004. Kindle edition. Excerpt. https://books.google.com/books?id=K-ZU35x2JaoC&pg=PA54&lpg=PA54&dq=How+much+did+government+spend+investigating+tylenol&source=bl&ots=MYVv0GgLiT&sig=aGgVsBpQN6ItG971z4EFlEjqaQ8&hl=en&sa=X&ved=0ahUKEwjBlLmwxrTMAhVDdj4KHQFKB00Q6AEILDAC#v=onepage&q=How%20much%20did%20government%20spend%20investigating%20tylenol&f=false.

Plante, Hank. "Reagan's Legacy." HIV Info—Hot Topics—from the Experts. San Francisco AIDS Foundation. 2011. http://sfaf.org/hiv-info/hot-topics/from-the-experts/2011-02-reagans-legacy.html?referrer=https://www.google.com/.

Reagan, Ronald. "The President's News Conference—September 17, 1985." https://reaganlibrary.archives.gov/archives/speeches/1985/91785c.htm.

Shoard, Catherine. "Elizabeth Taylor 'Worth up to 1Bn' at Time of Death." *Guardian*, March 29, 2011. http://www.theguardian.com/film/2011/mar/29/elizabeth-taylor-worth-1bn-death.

Stern, Mark Joseph. "Listen to Reagan's Press Secretary Laugh About Gay People Dying of AIDS." *Slate*, December 1, 2015. http://www.slate.com/blogs/outward/2015/12/01/reagan_press_secretary_laughs_about_gay_people_dying_of_aids.html.

Zweig, Stefan. *The World of Yesterday.* Lexington, MA: Plunkett Lake Press, 2011.

Acknowledgments

Writing the acknowledgments section in the book is one of the hardest parts for me, because pretty much everyone who has ever given me confidence was indispensible in writing this book. So, this book is for most everyone, but especially . . .

For Nicole Tourtelot, my wonderful agent. Without you I don't know where I would be, but, best-case scenario, probably writing lists about cats on the Internet. Thank you for saving me from that.

For Allison Adler, my brilliant first editor, who guided me through this process with so much kindness.

For Caroline Zancan, my second editor, who has fielded endless questions about this book.

Thanks to Kerry Cullen, an amazing editor who has patiently listened to me nit-pick over endless details.

For the people at Macmillan—it is still bizarre to me that there is a business model in letting me sit around and learn stuff and then tell stories about the stuff I learned, but I hope it is working out really well. It definitely is for me.

For Iris Smyles, who suggested the Dancing Plague *and* Encephalitis Lethargica. Thank you, and everyone should buy your book, *Dating Tips for the Unemployed*.

For Seth Porges, an endless font of ideas.

For The Hell's Belles, for making me laugh, always.

For Neesha Arter and Timothy Kuratek, for the photos and friendship.

For the women of Article Club, for giving me a space to yell about ideas.

For Lia Boyle, who patiently helped me understand the science behind these diseases.

For Sarah Maslin Nir, who had been a godmother to all my books.

For Peter Feld, who helped me get my first job when I came to New York.

For Chris Busch, who probably believed I was going to write a book before anyone.

For Dad, who, through endless childhood readings of Dave Barry and Mel Brooks viewings, taught me that you can make jokes about just about anything.

For Mom, who formatted the endnotes. Greater love hath no woman.

For Daniel, the ideal first reader, and the ideal mate. Every day I wonder how I got so lucky.

For Elizabeth Bielawska, a woman of incredible dignity. Daniel and I would be lost without your help.

For the Richard Family, who is handling death with such grace.

And for Sarah Richard: Beyond this place, there be dragons. I hope you're keeping them company until we join you.

Illustration Credits

All public domain except:

page

21   Column of Marcus Aurelius, Carole Raddato, Licensed under CC BY 2.0.
62   Free clipart, Last Word Larry, http://worldartsme.com/">WorldArtsMe</.
70   commons.wikimedia.org/wiki/User:Anthony92931, Licensed under CC BY SA-3.0.
90   Wellcome Images, Licensed under CC BY 4.0.
115 Wellcome Images, Licensed under CC BY 4.0.
123 flickr.com/photos/phyrephox, Licensed under CC BY SA-2.0.
140 Michael Billington, Licensed under CC BY SA-3.0.
238 flickr.com/photos/nostri-imago, Licensed under CC BY 2.0.
270 (bottom) Otis Historical Archives of "National Museum of Health & Medicine" (OTIS Archive 1), Licensed under CC BY 2.0.
271 (top left) WC585 1908R53d, "The Diagnosis of Smallpox," Ricketts, T. F, Casell and Company, 1908 Plate XXIV, Small child with smallpox showing an exceptional case because the trunk almost entirely escaped the invasion of smallpox, Licensed under CC by 4.0.
271 (top right) St Bartholomew's Hospital Archives & Museum, Wellcome Images, Licensed under CC by 4.0.
271 (bottom right) Wellcome Library, London, Licensed under CC BY 4.0.
272 (bottom right) The Bonkers Institute for Nearly Genuine Research, www.bonkersinstitute.org, Licensed under CC BY 3.0.

About the Author

JENNIFER WRIGHT is the author of *It Ended Badly: Thirteen of the Worst Breakups in History*. She has written for numerous publications, including *McSweeney's*, *The New York Observer*, *Salon*, *Cosmopolitan*, *Glamour*, *Popular Mechanics*, *Maxim*, *The New York Post*, and more. She lives in New York City with her fiancé, who is pretty sure she has a cold and not the bubonic plague.